The Rapid Fat Loss Handbook

A Scientific Approach to Crash Dieting

Lyle McDonald

This book is not intended for the treatment or prevention of disease, nor as a substitute for medical treatment, nor as an alternative to medical advice. It is a review of scientific evidence presented for information purposes only. Use of the guidelines herein is at the sole choice and risk of the reader.

Copyright:
First Edition © 2005 by Lyle McDonald. All rights reserved.
Second Edition © 2008 by Lyle McDonald. All rights reserved.

This book or any part thereof, may not be reproduced or recorded in any form without permission in writing from the publisher, except for brief quotations embodied in critical articles or reviews.

For information contact:
Lyle McDonald Publishing
PO Box 1713
Salt Lake City, Ut 84110
Email: lylemcd@comcast.net

Cover and interior book design by Jazz Kalsi
Email: jkalsi@gmail.com

ISBN: 978-0-9671456-4-8

SECOND EDITION
FIRST PRINTING

Acknowledgments

As always, I'd like to thank the members of my web forum for being both guinea pigs for the diet as well as providing invaluable feedback, especially on the final 4 chapters. A special thanks goes out to forum member Kurtis Thompson who helped me decide on a final book title.

And, of course I'd like to thank everybody who thinks enough of me to keep purchasing my books.

Table of Contents

Introduction

Just how quickly?...1

When is a crash diet appropriate?...7

Basic nutrition overview.. 11

Nutrient Metabolism Overview 17

An Overview of the Diet.. 21

Estimating body fat percentage... 25

Exercise... 39

Setting up the diet 43

Metabolic slowdown and what to do about it 55

Free meals, refeeds and diet breaks 63

Ending the Diet - Introduction 73

Moving to Maintenance: Non-counting Method Part 1 79

Moving to Maintenance: Non-counting Method Part 2 85

Moving to Maintenance: Calculation method... 95

Back To Dieting... 107

Appendix 1: BMI and Body fat charts... 113

My Other Books... 117

Introduction

I want to say at the outset that writing this book makes me a little bit uncomfortable for reasons I'll explain in a moment. Now, for the most part, an individual's personal choices are really none of my concern: what people do to or for themselves is their own problem. At the same time, I have a responsibility to my readers when I present something that has the potential to be harmful or damaging.

It's why I spent literally chapters discussing potential risks or side-effects in my previous books. Like the issue of dehydrating to make weight, crash dieting is a topic that I get a little bit antsy about. So why am I writing about it?

The first reason is reality. Trust me, I'd love to live in a world where nobody crash dieted, where everybody followed sane and safe dieting strategies and stuck with it in the long term until they reached their goal and then stuck with those newfound eating habits in the long-term. I also want a pony and to be six feet tall and to be an astronaut. And how about an end to world hunger while I'm at it. My point? When idealism and reality slam together it's never pretty. People are going to crash diet no matter what I or anybody else tell them.

Secondly, there are times when crash dieting might be more effective or even required. I know that mainstream nutritionist types will tell you that crash dieting is always bad but, as with just about any absolutist stance, this isn't necessarily correct. I'll talk about some of those situations in chapter two, times when crash dieting may be preferred or even required.

Finally, I am aware of at least two other approaches (Extreme Crash Dieting by Dr. Eric Serrano and The Radical Diet by Dr. Mauro DiPasquale) that address the issue of rapid weight and fat loss. I'm familiar with both books (and know both authors) and, well, being who and what I am, I know I can do better. I hope my readers feel the same.

The bottom line is this, no matter what I or anybody else says about it, people are going to crash diet. Sometimes it's necessary or beneficial, other times it's not. Regardless, people are going to do it. With that realization made, I figure that the least that can be done is to make sure that such crash diets are done as safely and as intelligently as possible. Using nutritional science and research, we can develop a crash diet that isn't totally stupid, that will be safe and sane (within the limits of crash dieting) at least compared to everything else that's out there.

Trust me, there's a lot of really dumb ways to lose weight fast out there. All vegetables, all fruit, nothing but broth, that cabbage soup thing, just a lot of stupid, stupid stuff. This book isn't such an approach. It relies on cutting edge nutritional science to ensure that rapid weight/fat loss is accomplished as effectively and safely as possible. I'd be lying if I said it was an easy diet, but it is an effective one.

The obligatory warning

Now matter how safe you make it, extended crash dieting can cause problems, both physiologically and psychologically (I'll talk about each in a later chapter). I'm going to be very specific in terms of the time frames I think people should use such an extreme approach. I'm not kidding when I say that you should follow them. Frankly, that's really my main concern about writing this book: I understand human behavior when it comes to this stuff.

People tend to read diet books selectively, hearing what they want to hear and ignoring the rest (especially the warnings). Once people hear just how much fat they can lose in a short period of time, they lose their minds. They'll try to stay on an extreme approach like this for extended periods of time and get themselves into trouble. Then they blame me. And I simply don't need that in my life. If you're not going to follow my recommendations exactly, don't blame anyone but yourself if you get into problems. My recommendations are going to be very specific, you ignore them at your own risk.

Just how quickly

I've started my last two books with a chapter (or five) addressing a specific problem, then working to what I consider the solution. I'm going to spare you that endless verbiage this time and jump right into the main topic. Since this is a book about rapid weight/fat loss and crash dieting, I imagine all of my readers want to know just how quickly weight and/or fat can be lost. Before I can answer that question (and even to clear up what I suspect may be some confusion by my readers on the previous sentence), I have to cover a bit of physiology first.

Weight versus fat: They are not the same thing

Every tissue in your body (including muscle, body fat, your heart, liver, spleen, kidneys, bones, etc.) weighs a given amount. We could (conceivably anyhow) take them out of your body, plop them on a scale and find out how much they weigh. Your total *body weight* is comprised of the weight of every one of those tissues. But only some percentage of your total body *weight* is body *fat*.

Researchers and techie types frequently divide the body into two (or more) components including fat mass (the sum total of the body fat you have on your body) and lean body mass (everything else). I don't want to get into a bunch of technical details regarding different types of body fat.

Let's say that we could magically determine the weight of only your fat cells. Of course, we know your total weight by throwing you on a scale. By dividing the total amount of fat into the total body weight, you can determine a body fat percentage which represents the percentage of your total weight that is fat.

Lean athletes might only carry 5-10% body fat, meaning that only 5-10% of their total weight is fat. A 200-pound athlete with 10% body fat is carrying 20 pounds (200 * 0.10 =

20) of body fat. The remaining 180 pounds (200 total pounds - 20 pounds of fat = 180 pounds) of weight is muscle, organs, bones, water, etc. Researchers call the remaining 180 pounds lean body mass or LBM. I'll be using LBM a lot so make sure and remember what it means: LBM is lean body mass, the amount of your body that is not fat.

In cases of extreme obesity, a body fat percentage of 40-50% or higher is not unheard of. Meaning that nearly one-half of that person's total weight is fat. A 400-pound person with 50% body fat is carrying 200 pounds of body fat. The other 200 pounds is muscle, organs, bones, etc. Again, that's 200 pounds of LBM.

Most people fall somewhere between the two extremes described above. An average male may carry from 18-23% body fat and an average female somewhere between 25-30% body fat. A male at 180 pounds and 20% body fat is carrying 36 pounds of fat and the rest of his weight (180 pounds – 36 pounds = 144 pounds) is LBM. A 150-pound female at 30% body fat has 50 pounds of body fat and 100 pounds of LBM.

I bring this up as many (if not most) diet books focus only on weight loss, without making the above distinction. I should note that more current books have finally started to distinguish between *fat* loss and *weight* loss.

Why is this important?

So let's say you start a diet, reducing some part of your daily food intake. Maybe you start exercising as well. After some time period, you get on the scale and it says you've lost ten pounds. That's 10 pounds of *weight*. But how much of it is *fat*? Frankly, you have no way of knowing with just the scale (unless it's one of those Tanita body fat scales, which attempt to estimate body fat percentage but which tend not to be terribly accurate).

You could have lost fat or muscle or just dropped a lot of water. Even a big bowel movement can cause a *weight* loss of a pound or two (or more, depending). A colonic that clears out your entire lower intestinal tract may cause a significant weight loss. The scale can't tell you what you've lost, it can only tell you how much you have lost.

When you're worrying about long-term changes, the real goal is *fat* loss (some LBM loss is occasionally acceptable but that's more detail than I want to get into here). That is, cycling water weight on and off of your body (as frequently happens with certain dieting approaches) isn't really moving you towards any real goal even if it makes you think you are. Don't get me wrong, it may be beneficial in the short-term (again, I'll talk about reasons to crash diet shortly) but it doesn't represent true *fat* loss.

My point in bringing up this distinction is that it's easy to hide the true results of a diet by not making the distinction between *weight* loss and *fat* loss. In many diets, and in the case of the crash diet I'm going to describe, total *weight* loss will drastically outstrip true *fat* loss. As above, this may have benefits or not but I wanted to make sure everyone was clear coming out of the gate. I also don't want to get accused of misleading my readers by making them think that the total *weight* loss is all *fat* loss; it's not.

Just how quickly?

So just how quickly can you lose fat (or weight for that matter)? Most mainstream diet books and authorities echo the idea that two pounds per week (a little less than one kilogram per week for the metrically inclined) is the maximum. Where did this value come from? Frankly, I have no idea.

To at least some degree, it probably represents about the maximum weight/fat loss that most feel *should* be attempted. To understand this, I have to do a little bit of math for you. One pound of fat contains roughly 3,500 calories of energy. Therefore to lose two pounds of fat per week (this assumes that you are losing 100% fat which is usually a poor assumption) requires that you create a weekly deficit of 7,000 calories.

This means that you either have to restrict your food intake or increase your energy expenditure (with exercise or drugs) by that much. Obviously, that averages out to 1,000 calories per day. You either end up having to restrict food pretty severely or have to engage in hours of exercise each day. From that perspective alone, losing faster than two pounds per week is considered unrealistic or unwise.

At the same time, it's not uncommon to see claims of weight losses of one pound per day or three to five pounds per week on some diets. In the initial stages of some diets, weight losses of 15-20 pounds are not unheard of. Are these all lies? Not exactly. Part of it has to do with the issue of *weight* loss and *fat* loss discussed above. An extremely large individual, put on a restrictive diet can probably lose significantly more than two pounds of *weight* per week. But it won't all be *fat*.

This is especially true for the myriad low-carbohydrate dieting approaches out there. Studies demonstrate a rapid weight loss of anywhere from 1-15 pounds in the first week or two of a low-carbohydrate diet and average weight losses of 7-10 pounds in the first week are fairly standard. Most of it is simply water loss although some of it will be true tissue loss, meaning fat and muscle. After that initial rapid weight loss, true weight/fat loss slows down to more "normal" levels.

The same goes in reverse, by the way, when you take someone on a low-carbohydrate diet and feed them carbs again, it's not uncommon to see weight spike by many pounds very quickly. A high salt intake can cause a rather large retention of water (especially if you've been on a low-salt diet) and most women will readily tell you about the rapid weight gain (from water retention) that occurs during their menstrual cycle.

Why does it matter?

I bring this up for the simple reason that the diet I'm going to describe is going to cause both rapid weight **and** fat losses. Just realize that the total weight loss (which may range from 10-20 pounds over 2 weeks) isn't all comprised of body fat and I don't want to play the rather intellectually dishonest game of making you think it does. A majority of it is going to be water loss. As discussed next chapter, this isn't *necessarily* a bad thing.

Diet overview

Though I'll give you many more details in an upcoming chapter, the diet described in this book is a slightly modified version of a dietary approach called a protein sparing modified fast (PSMF). The original PSMF was a very low calorie diet consisting of lean proteins (amounts varying depending on specific circumstances), a small amount of fat and carbohydrate, some vegetables (and other zero-calorie foods), some basic supplements, and nothing else.

Quick tangent: Didn't some people die?

Older dieters or just historians of the field may remember that there were some deaths in the late 70's and early 80's in individuals following something called The Last Chance Diet. This particular diet was a protein sparing modified fast centered on supplemental liquid nutrition but the folks who developed the product couldn't have done a worse job in designing it. First they picked the cheapest protein source available, collagen: a protein that provides essentially zero nutrition to the body.

Second, they provided no supplemental vitamins and minerals (some of which would have been obtained if the dieters had been eating whole foods in the first place). This caused a couple of problems including the loss of heart muscle (from the total lack of protein) and cardiac arrhythmias from the lack of minerals. Basically, the problem wasn't with the approach so much as with the terrible food choices. PSMFs based around whole foods (which provide high quality proteins as well as vitamins and minerals) and with adequate mineral supplementation have shown no such problems.

What can you expect?

On average, caloric intakes on this diet will come out to between 400 to 1200 calories per day coming almost exclusively from protein. For those of you familiar with ketogenic (low-carbohydrate, high-fat) diets, a PSMF is essentially a ketogenic diet without the dietary fat. Obviously, this will represent a fairly large caloric deficit; how large depending on your starting body weight and activity levels.

So with all of that in mind, you may still be wondering what you can expect in terms of true fat loss per week. A lot of it, actually, will depend on where you're starting out body weight wise (activity also factors in), as that determines your maintenance caloric level.

A 165-pound male with normal activity patterns may have a maintenance requirement of about 2700 calories per day. At 800 calories per day on this diet, that's almost a 2000 calorie per day deficit, 14,000 calories over a week, 28,000 calories over 2 weeks (note: there is a slowing of metabolic rat that reduces these values somewhat). Assuming all of the true (non-water) weight lost was fat (it won't be), that should be an 8-pound fat loss in 2 weeks (28,000 / 3,500 = 8) or approximately 2/3rd of a pound of fat lost per day. The true fat loss will be lower because of various inefficiencies and the slowdown of metabolic rate (which can start after only 3-4 days of severe caloric restriction).

A larger individual, say 250 pounds, may have a maintenance caloric requirement near 3,750 calories per day. At 800 cal per day on this diet, that's a 3,000-calorie per day deficit. Over 2 weeks, that's a 42,000-calorie deficit, divided by 3,500 calories per pound of fat equals 12 pounds of fat.   That's on top of the 10 or more pounds of water that may be lost.

Females or lighter individuals with their generally lower maintenance caloric requirements will lose less. True fat losses of 1/2 pound per day or slightly less may be all that they get: that still amounts to a considerable fat loss (6-7 pounds true fat loss over 2 weeks) along with the extra water weight loss.

The bottom line being that an approach such as the crash diet can take off both fat and weight far more rapidly than less extreme diets. And while I still think it's generally better for dieters to take the long-approach and use less extreme diets for longer periods of time, as I'll discuss in the next chapter, under some circumstances, crash dieting can be beneficial.

6

When is a crash diet appropriate?

As mentioned in the introduction, there are a number of situations that might warrant a crash diet and I want to discuss those in this chapter. Then, after two quick chapters of basic nutrition physiology, I'll get into the brass tacks (what does that phrase mean anyway?) of doing the diet.

I want to make the point again that, in almost all of the situations I'm going to describe, my ideal is that individuals take the sane and slow approach to fat loss, set up a reasonable diet, lose weight/fat over an extended period until they reach their goals. As per the introduction, when idealism and reality collide, it gets ugly and there are situations where crash dieting is necessary, preferred or simply required. I may have missed one or two situations but I think I cover all of them below.

An upcoming special event

I imagine many women and men reading this book can relate to the concept of an upcoming special event like a wedding or high school reunion where they feel the need to drop weight (and some fat) rapidly: either to impress old schoolmates or to fit into a special outfit for the occasion. People have suggested that I remarket this book as "The Desperate Bride's Rapid Fat Loss Diet" for exactly that reason.

Similarly, models or actors, whose income often requires that they maintain (or at least reach) a certain shape or weight, could get into a situation where they needed rapid results. Often a great deal of money (gained or lost) rests on the ability to do so.

The simple reality is that, even if it would have been better to start your diet months ago and take a moderate, long-term approach to fat and weight loss, that isn't always possible. Time crunch require desperate measures. A 10-20 pound total weight loss including a four to seven pounds of true fat loss can help to get them in shape for the occasion.

Kickstarting a more moderate diet

Using a short crash-diet to kickstart a more moderate/long-term approach to fat loss may be one of the best uses of what's described in this book. Frankly, one of the bigger problems associated with the long slow approach to dieting is that people get frustrated with the rate of weight loss: it's always slower than they want it to be.

Seriously, if someone is losing one pound per week, they want to lose two, if they are losing two pounds per week, they want to lose four. If they were losing ten pounds per week, they'd want to lose 20. And after seeing some of the absolutely amazing losses on shows like "The Biggest Loser", they probably want to know how they can lose 30 pounds in a week. In any case, you get the idea. Chalk it up to normal human behavior, the "immediate gratification" society we live in or whatever explanation makes you happiest.

Frankly, I don't care why people think this way; I simply know that they do. By starting with a few weeks of crash dieting, weight loss is kick started and this can give the necessary positive reinforcement needed to keep folks moving ahead. As well, since the crash diet described here is based around whole foods (many approaches are geared around various supplements and powdered drinks), it helps with the initial stages of food reeducation. By gradually increasing intake of "better" foods on top of what the crash diet already contains, dieters can get on the track to making permanent changes in their eating habits. I'll come back to this when I talk about ending a crash diet.

Contest bodybuilders

Contest bodybuilding is as much a test of extreme willpower as of anything else. Frankly, it's not healthy to starve the body down to such super low body fat percentages. But, as it is part of the sport to be this lean, it is a necessary evil.

Normally, contest bodybuilders will follow a progressively more restrictive diet starting 12 or more weeks out from their show. However, sometimes they get behind schedule and need to get caught up. Maybe they were fatter than they thought to begin with, maybe it's their first show and they don't know their body well enough, maybe their coach is just an incompetent. Any number of things can throw off a contest diet and getting into shape sometimes takes extreme measures. Ten to 14 days of crash dieting can get a bodybuilder back on track, or at least closer to making contest shape.

Other weight class athletes/other athletes

Although bodybuilders lose extreme amounts of fat (and frequently dehydrate) for appearance reasons, many athletes have to do the same to make it into their weight class (or simply to perform better). Some examples are wrestlers, powerlifters and Olympic lifters, etc. Although it would be far better for such an athlete to keep their true weight closer to their goal and just dehydrate slightly to make it in, that doesn't always happen. Sometimes weight class athletes have to drop a tremendous amount of weight (and the more fat they can drop, the less they have to dehydrate) quickly.

Other athletes may also have a need to drop fat/weight quickly to improve their performance. Think about an endurance athlete who may improve their power to weight ratio by dropping weight or someone of that nature. I should note, and I'll come back to this, that dehydration beyond even a small level can really destroy performance capacity (extreme dehydration can cause death) so the crash diet should be used several weeks prior to the main event to drop a few pounds of fat such that normal hydration can be reattained before competition.

Other applications

I'm sure creative readers can think of other possible times when a crash diet approach might be valid or appropriate. One that comes to mind is the case where someone has to have surgery and needs to drop weight rapidly for it to be done safely. I simply want to point out that anyone in that situation must be medically monitored during the diet phase and shouldn't be using this or any other diet book to self-prescribe a diet.

A very common usage of the rapid fat loss program among members of my forum (http://www.bodyrecomposition.com/forums) is to simply get the dieting phase over with faster. Folks would simply rather diet hard for a couple of weeks and get the fat off then take the month or more that it would take with a more conventional diet. This allows them to get back to other goals (such as strength or muscle mass gains) as quickly as possible.

10

Basic nutrition overview

Since I can't assume what level of knowledge readers of this book have, I want to give a very brief overview of human nutrition. And when I say brief, I mean brief. In total, I want to address the major categories of nutrients, talk about what they are used for in the body, and give examples of some of the major food sources of each.

Essential and nonessential nutrients

The body has a daily requirement for somewhere around 60 nutrients on a daily basis for normal functioning (note: as nutritional science has progressed, it's now become apparent that many, many more nutrients may provide optimal health, although they are not necessarily required for life). This includes substances such as air and water that, while they aren't considered as nutrients per se, are usually not an issue.

Of more relevance to this book, nutritional science often groups nutrients into the categories of essential and nonessential (recently the terms indispensable and dispensable have come into vogue) which is what I'd like to discuss next. Summarizing, there are roughly 8 essential amino acids, 2 essential fatty acids, a host of vitamins and minerals and a few others substances that are required on a daily basis. You'll note that I didn't list carbohydrate as one of the essential nutrients mainly because, well, it's not essential. I'll come back to this below.

I want to make it clear that the term nonessential doesn't mean that the nutrient isn't essential for human health; rather it isn't essential to obtain the nutrient from the diet. Translating that into English, there are some nutrients (such as glucose, some fatty acids, and about half of the amino acids) that can be made in the body from other sources. They are essential for life but it is not essential that you obtain them from your diet.

At the same time, there are nutrients that cannot be made by the body (the vitamins and minerals are examples, so are the essential fatty acids and roughly the other half of the amino acids) and are hence considered essential nutrients. That is, it is essential that they

11

be obtained from the diet. I want to make it clear that this is a vast simplification of the concept but I don't want to get into nit picky details that are unnecessary for this book.

I bring it up mainly because the diet I'm going to describe in this book is built around the concept of decreasing food intake to include *only* the essential nutrients. That is, the goal of the diet is to provide only the essential nutrients, while removing everything that is nonessential, in order to generate the greatest caloric deficit and the most rapid weight/fat loss possible. I'll note that, since the diet is based around whole foods, there will be an intake of the nonessential amino acids along with the essential aminos. While it very well might be conceivable to structure the rapid fat loss plan around a supplement which only provided the essential amino acids, in the long-run this would do nothing to help with long-term food consumption patterns. It also would be terribly unsatisfying and unfulfilling.

So with that basic overview, let's look at the major nutrient categories: protein, carbohydrates, fat, fiber and alcohol.

Protein

The word protein come from a Greek word meaning "the first" which is meant to signify its primary role in human nutrition. As I'll discuss in some detail in the next chapter, while the body can survive fairly extended periods without any carbohydrates or fat, a lack of protein leads to a loss of body tissue (muscle and organ protein), function and eventually death.

So what is protein? Dietary proteins are made up of compounds called amino acids, of which ~20 occur in the diet (there are many more that occur in the body). Of those, about half are considered essential meaning that they must come from the diet. Under certain conditions, such as stress and trauma, some amino acids also become conditionally essential but this isn't that important to this book.

Proteins have a number of crucial roles in the human body but most of them are structural (meaning the protein is used to build things). Many hormones are made of protein, your organs, muscles, skin and hair are made of protein; protein has several other roles in the body as well. Something to note is that, in contrast to carbohydrate (which is stored in both muscle and liver) and fat (which is stored on your ass and stomach), there is no real storage form of protein unless you count the small amount floating around in the bloodstream and the protein that makes up your muscles and organs (which you generally don't want to break down for other uses). This has implications for dieting (and starvation) that I'll discuss in the next chapter.

Protein is found to some degree in almost all foods with the exception of pure fats like vegetable oils and such and some totally refined carbohydrates such as candy (e.g. jelly beans). Fruits and vegetables contain fairly small amounts of protein (perhaps a gram or two per serving) while beans and nuts contain significant amounts of protein. But most people in modern society get their protein from animal based products: meat (red meat,

12

chicken, fish), milk, cheeses, etc. Since I imagine most readers are familiar with calories (joules in non-US countries), I want to mention that protein contains 4 calories per gram.

Carbohydrate

Without getting into the current controversy over carbohydrates in the human diet, I'll simply point out again that there is no strict nutritional requirement for carbohydrate. This is true for a couple of reasons that I'll discuss in the next chapter.

First, I want to subdivide carbohydrates into two general categories: starchy and fibrous (this is a common bodybuilding/athletic method of differentiating them even if it's a bit simplistic). Fibrous carbohydrates are all your high-fiber carbs, meaning vegetables (i.e. the foods most people don't like to eat). With a few exceptions, noted below, they tend to contain very little digestible carbohydrate while simultaneously containing a good bit of fiber.

Starchy carbohydrates are, more or less, everything else: breads, pasta, rice, and grains, basically any carbohydrate that contains a good bit of digestible carbohydrate. I should note that there are a few starchy vegetables such as carrots, peas, corn and potatoes: vegetables which contain larger amount of digestible carbohydrate and which should be counted as starchy carbohydrates in terms of tallying up daily carbohydrate intake. Fruits, while not technically a starch, would be included in that category since they contain quite a bit of digestible carbohydrate.

Explaining the caloric value of carbohydrates can be somewhat confusing. Starchy carbohydrates contain 4 calories per gram but since you won't be eating any of these on this diet, that's sort of an irrelevant point (it will become important when you read about moving to maintenance, the full diet break, and other topics discussed later in this book).

You've probably heard that the human body can't derive any calories from fiber but this isn't entirely true, various bacteria in your gut breaks down fiber into compounds that your body can use and fiber has been given a rough approximate caloric value of 1.5-2 calories/gram. Unless you're consuming an absolute ton of it per day, you can generally ignore the caloric value of fiber. For example, a daily intake of 25 grams of fiber would only contribute ~40-50 calories/day to the diet.

In the body, carbohydrate is only used as a fuel. Incoming dietary carbohydrates are either used immediately for energy, stored for later (as glycogen in the muscle and liver) or, under fairly rare conditions, converted to fat and stored. All tissues of the body can use glucose (which is what all dietary carbohydrates eventually get broken down to after digestion and absorption) and most will use it when it is available.

At the same time, with a few exceptions, those same tissues will happily use fatty acids (from either the diet or the fat stored on your body) for fuel when carbohydrates are not available. I should note that carbohydrates (stored as glycogen in the muscle) are necessary to support high intensity exercise such as weight training or sprinting. I'll address this issue in a later chapter.

Fat and cholesterol

Even though they are chemically and nutritionally distinct substances, fat and cholesterol are so linked in the minds of most people that I'm going to discuss them in the same section.

Dietary fat can be used directly for energy and also plays a variety of structural roles in the body (it is used in cell membranes and some hormones are made out of cholesterol; a class of compounds called the eicosanoids are made out of specific fatty acids). Fundamentally, that's what body fat is, stored fat that provides energy to your body when you aren't eating enough (or you're exercising or starving or what have you). When you are "losing fat", you are mobilizing stored fatty acids from your fat cells and burning them for energy elsewhere.

Although there can be very slight differences, practically speaking all fats are given the same value which is 9 calories per gram. However, it appears that different fats have a slightly different tendency to be stored as body fat. Since you'll only be consuming a very small amount of dietary fat, and that will come from the omega-3s (discussed below) anyhow, this is an irrelevancy for this diet. Cholesterol isn't used for energetic purposes and has no caloric value for humans.

The biggest controversies regarding dietary fat usually revolve around the health effects of its consumption. It's not unfair to say that, for many years now, dietary fat has been the whipping boy of the nutritional world (though carbohydrates are taking that role in recent years): fat makes you fat, fat causes heart disease and cancer, fat is probably responsible for terrorism in the US and the decline in the family unit. You name it and the problem has probably been blamed on dietary fat. Cholesterol intake (which, often but not always, accompanies fat intake) shares a similar negative reputation. As with so many extremist stances, the truth is a little different.

First and foremost is the fact that, except in a fairly small percentage of people, dietary cholesterol has little to no impact on blood cholesterol levels. Quite in fact, your body (your liver to be exact) generally makes more cholesterol than you eat in a day. Additionally, your liver will modify how much cholesterol it produces depending on your daily intake. If your cholesterol intake goes up, your liver makes less; if cholesterol intake goes down, your liver makes more. Your body is smart that way.

Rather, the types and amounts of dietary fat being consumed play a far larger role in blood lipid levels. Frankly, I don't have much more to say about dietary cholesterol, it's simply not that big of a deal unless you are in that small percentage of folks who are sensitive to it.

So let's talk some more about fat or rather triglycerides, which is what constitutes most of your daily fat intake. In the past ten years or so, the issue of fat quality (i.e. type of fat) has become just as important as that of fat quantity (i.e. amount of fat). Simply put: all fats are not the same in terms of their effects on health.

The four main categories of fats are discussed next.

Trans-fatty acids

Trans-fatty acids are a man-made fat made by bubbling hydrogen through vegetable oil to make it semisolid with a long-shelf life. Margarine is probably the example most readers are familiar with although trans-fatty acids (also called partially hydrogenated vegetable oils) are found in almost all processed foods. Of all the fats, trans-fatty acids have the worst effect on blood lipids and overall health. Their high prevalence in the modern diet is likely a large contributor to at least some of our modern health problems and they have no place in this or any other diet.

Saturated fats

Saturated fats are found almost exclusively in animal products (two exceptions are coconut and palm kernel oil) and are solid at room temperature. Think butter or the solid fat found on the rim of a steak. The impact of saturated fats turns out to be much more complicated than simply "saturated fats are bad". Some saturated fats raise blood cholesterol while others have absolutely no effect. Regardless, as they are not essential to human life (not to mention that there are plenty stored in your body fat already), saturated fats are not included on this diet.

Monounsaturated fat

Monounsaturates are present in almost all foods which contain fat and are liquid at room temperature. Olive oil is a major source of monounsaturated fats and has received a great deal of attention as a relatively healthy fat. Monounsaturates have a neutral, if not beneficial, effect on health and it's thought that the high olive oil consumption among Mediterraneans is partly responsible for their robust health. Although healthy, monounsaturated fats are not essential and not part of this diet.

Polyunsaturated fats

Polyunsaturated fats are found primarily in vegetable oils and are liquid at room temperature. They are generally claimed to have a positive effect on human health although, as always, things are a little more complicated than that.

Polyunsaturated fats come in two major "flavors", referred to as omega-three and omega-6 fatty acids. The omega-3 fatty acids include the fish oils which I imagine most have at least heard about. Without going into huge amounts of detail, I bring up the distinction because excess omega-6 can be harmful to health, especially if the intake of omega-3 is low. This is especially true in the modern diet where omega-6 intake vastly outstrips omega-3 intake.

The key thing for readers to realize is that omega-3 fatty acids are the real nutritional powerhouses with the fish oils (EPA and DHA, you don't want to know the full names, trust me on this) having a profoundly beneficial effect on human health and fat loss. If I listed all of the known good effects of fish oils, you'd think I was making it up but the research is there. On the rapid fat loss diet, outside of the small amounts of fat found in the foods you'll be eating, the omega-3's should be about the only fat you consume. Pre-formed fish oils or liquid fish oil are both acceptable sources.

In the first edition of this book, I also allowed for flaxseed oil as another potential source of omega-3 fatty acids; this is no longer the case. Recent research has established that the conversion of flaxseed oil to EPA and DHA is completely inefficient and ineffective in humans, flaxseed does little to raise the body's EPA levels and nothing to raise DHA levels. For dieters who dislike swallowing pills, a liquid fish oil product such as Carlson's is my recommendation.

Everything else: Fiber, alcohol, vitamins and minerals

Fiber is not considered an essential nutrient but it plays many important roles in human health. Fiber can be subdivided into two major (and several minor) categories which are soluble and insoluble fiber. Soluble fibers mix in water and take up a lot of space in the stomach: this is good while dieting as it increases feelings of fullness. Insoluble fibers don't mix with water but help with bowel regularity and keep the colon healthy (fiber: it's nature's broom). Both are important to human health and both are found in varying degrees in vegetables and fruits (and, of course, fiber supplements).

Alcohol really isn't a nutrient in that it provides nothing of nutritional value (except maybe energy) to the body. It provides calories and alters nutrient metabolism in a fashion that tends to promote fat gain. While it would be ridiculous to say that alcohol has no place on any diet, it certainly has no place on the diet described in this book.

Finally, there are the vitamins and minerals which serve hundreds, if not thousands, of roles in the human body. Minerals like calcium, for example, are not only structural (bone is mainly calcium) but are also involved in cellular signaling. Vitamins act as nutritional cofactors for enzymes and are simply necessary for the body to function optimally. Vitamins and minerals are found in varying amounts in the food supply with fruit and vegetables being a key provider.

As well, a class of nutrients called phytochemicals are found only in vegetables and are currently thought to provide many health benefits to the body. The various antioxidants (which help to protect cells from damage) are found in varying amounts throughout the food supply with fruits and vegetables being key sources.

Nutrient Metabolism Overview

In this chapter, I want to give readers a very brief and simplified overview of human metabolism and nutrient use. Which, for those who know a lot about the topic will realize, is an understatement of vast proportion. The complexities of human metabolism can and do fill up hundreds of pages in physiology books and this chapter should be taken with that in mind.

The basics: Energy and building blocks

Very simplistically speaking, we can divide the uses of the nutrients (discussed last chapter) into three categories, of which I only really want to talk about two. One category, which I won't discuss much has to do with the vitamins and minerals which both act, essentially, as nuts and bolts in the body. They fulfill any number of different roles; depending on which one you're talking about. While critical to human health, they simply aren't that important to the topic of this book. If you're interested, go get yourself a book on vitamins and minerals and go to town. All I'm going to say is that you should make an effort to ensure your vitamin and mineral intake. A basic one-per-day multivitamin should probably be good "nutritional insurance" for everyone, the obsessed can look at versions containing mega-doses or what have you of the different nutrients.

The second category is for use as building blocks. Most parts of the human body are in a constant state of breakdown and buildup and nutrients must come in to the body to provide building blocks for those processes. One I imagine all readers are familiar with is that of calcium (a mineral) being the building block for bones. Additionally, skeletal muscle, organs and many hormones have amino acids (coming from protein) as their building blocks. As well, both fats and cholesterol play a role as a building block for cell membranes and a few other substances in the body.

The third category, and the one I'll spend the most time on in this chapter, is as an energy (fuel) source. Even as you sit reading this and growing bored, your body is using energy at some rate. So your brain, your heart and other organs, skeletal muscle, liver and even your fat cells are using energy, although the rates at which each uses energy varies from high (e.g. brain, liver) to extremely low (e.g. fat cells). Surprisingly and quite contrary to common belief, at rest skeletal muscle doesn't burn that many calories. The idea that adding muscle mass will turn you into a calorie burning inferno is simply incorrect.

Where does the energy come from?

So where does that energy come from? At the lowest level of cellular function, the only form of energy that your cells can use directly is something called adenosine triphosphate (ATP). I doubt that factoid is very helpful to readers except perhaps as the answer to a Trivial Pursuit or game show question. If you happen to sit around having polite conversation about ATP, please send me an email: I want to hang out with you.

Of more use to us, the body generates ATP from the burning (oxidation or combustion to use a more sciency term) of either glucose from carbohydrate or fatty acids from fats. Under specific circumstances protein can be used to produce ATP, either directly or via the conversion to either glucose or fat (usually protein is converted to glucose to be used for fuel). I'll come back to this below.

With a few exceptions that I'll talk about in a second, every tissue in your body can use either carbohydrate or fat for fuel. What determines which they use? For the most part, it's the availability of carbohydrates: when carbs are available (because you're eating plenty of them), those tissues will use carbohydrates, in the form of glucose, for fuel. When carbs are not available (because you're restricting them), the body will switch to using fat for fuel. That fat can either come from your diet or from the fat stored on your butt or stomach. This has another implication that is often forgotten in weight/fat reduction programs: when you eat more carbohydrates, your body uses less fat for energy; when you eat less carbohydrates, your body uses more fat for energy.

So what about those exceptions? A few tissues in your body such as the brain/central nervous system and one or two others can't use fatty acids for fuel; they can only use glucose. The brain is the main one I want to talk about here. It's usually (and incorrectly) stated that the brain can only use glucose for fuel, and this is true if you only consider glucose, amino acids, and fat as potential fuel sources. But this leaves out a fourth, extremely important, fuel source: ketones (also known as ketone bodies). Ketones are made from the breakdown of fat in the liver and function as a fat-derived fuel for the brain during periods of starvation/carbohydrate restriction.

I'll talk about starvation in more detail in a second but I want to mention that, after a few weeks in ketosis (a state where ketones build up in the bloodstream such that fuels such as the brain start using them for energy), the brain can derive 75% of its total energy from ketone metabolism. The other 25% comes from glucose.

So aren't carbohydrates essential?

At this point you may be slightly confused about the role of carbohydrates in the diet. In the last chapter, I stated that carbohydrates weren't an essential nutrient and above I mentioned that a few tissues can only use glucose and that even the brain gets about 25% of its total fuel requirements from glucose after adaptation to ketosis. So if those tissues still require glucose for energy, you may be wondering how carbohydrates aren't essential in the diet. Remember from the last chapter what the two requirements of an essential nutrient are:

1. That nutrient is required for the proper function of the body.

2. The body can't make that nutrient in sufficient quantities.

The second criterion is the reason that dietary carbohydrate is not an essential nutrient: the body is able to make as much glucose as the brain and the few other tissues need on a day-to-day basis. I should mention that the body is not able to provide sufficient carbohydrate to fuel high intensity exercise such as sprinting or weight training and carbs might be considered essential for individuals who want to do that type of exercise.

So how is the glucose made? The answer is a biochemical process with the unwieldy name of gluconeogenesis, which simply means the making of new glucose. This process primarily occurs in the liver. When necessary, the body can make glucose out of a number of other substances including glycerol (which comes from fat metabolism), lactate and pyruvate (which comes from carbohydrate metabolism), and certain amino acids (from protein).

Which brings me back around to the topic of protein as a fuel source for the body. Readers may have read that "carbohydrates spare protein" and this is part of the basis for that claim: when carbohydrates are being eaten in sufficient quantities, the body has no need to break down protein for fuel. By extension, when carbohydrates are being restricted for whatever reason, some proportion of protein will be used to make glucose, leaving less to be used for building blocks. This has an important implication for dieting, namely that protein requirements go up when you're restricting either calories or carbohydrates.

What about starvation?

Now seems like as good of a time to talk about starvation, the consumption of zero food. I should mention that therapeutic starvation (as it was called) was tried during the middle of the 20th century for weight loss, frequently causing rather rapid losses of weight. But it had an unfortunate problem, which I'm going to address below. For now, let's look at starvation and what happens.

So let's say you stop eating anything and look at what happens (a much more detailed examination of this and many other topics can be found in my first book The Ketogenic Diet). Over the first few hours of starvation, blood glucose and insulin levels both drop. This signals the body to break down glycogen (stored carbohydrate) in the liver to release it into the bloodstream. As well, the body starts mobilizing fat from fat cells to use for fuel. After 12-18 hours or so (faster if you exercise), liver glycogen is emptied. At this point blood glucose will drop to low-normal levels and stay there. Blood fatty acids will have increased significantly by this point.

After a day or so, most cells in the body, with a few exceptions, are using fatty acids for fuel. Obese individuals may derive over 90% of their total fuel requirements from fat while leaner individuals may only derive about 75% of the total from fat. So far so good, right, the body is mobilizing and utilizing an absolute ton of fatty acids for fuel: 90% of your total energy expenditure if you're fat and 75% if you're lean (I'll talk about what fat and lean is in another chapter).

There must be a drawback and here it is: the few tissues that require glucose are getting it via gluconeogenesis in the liver. As above, gluconeogenesis occurs from glycerol, lactate, pyruvate and amino acids. Now, if the person isn't eating any protein, where are those amino acids going to have to come from?

That's right, from the protein that is already in the body. But recall from last chapter that there really isn't a store of protein in the body, unless you count muscles and organs. Which means that, during total starvation, the body has to break down protein tissues to provide amino acids to make glucose. The body starts eating its own lean body mass to make glucose to fuel certain tissues. This is bad.

Now, as fatty acids start to accumulate and be burned in the liver, ketones will start to be produced. Initially, for reasons totally unimportant to this book, muscles will use the majority of ketones that are produced. As I mentioned above, after a few weeks, the brain will adapt so that it is using ketones and deriving most of its fuel from them; the small remainder comes from the glucose being produced via gluconeogenesis.

Now, the adaptation to ketosis occurs for a profoundly important reason. Once again, much of the glucose produced in the body is from amino acids which are coming from the protein in muscle (and to a lesser degree, organs). If such a breakdown continued in the long term, so much muscle would be lost that the individual who was starving would be unable to move. Quite in fact, the loss of too much lean body mass (muscle and organs) causes death. The shift to using ketones decreases the need to break down body protein to make glucose.

As I mentioned above, therapeutic starvation was often used in the cases where rapid weight loss was needed. And while it did generate rather high levels of weight and fat loss, it had as a problem the loss of excessive body protein. So researchers decided to find a way to try and generate similar levels of weight/fat loss while sparing LBM. And that's the topic of the next chapter.

An Overview of the Diet

Most diet books spend chapters selling you on a diet which generally only takes about a page or so (three pages if it's particularly complicated) to actually describe. That's followed with food lists and meal plans and it's not unfair to say that your average 300 page diet book will consist of 8 chapters selling you on it, a few pages describing the diet, and 150 pages of food lists and recipes.

I prefer to take a different approach; I spend chapters boring you to death with underlying physiology before actually describing the diet which often takes about a page or so. If nothing else, even if you never use the dietary advice, at least I figure that you've learned something valuable. That's what I've done in this book anyhow although please realize how much wasted verbiage I've spared you by avoiding unnecessary details. While I don't do meal plans, I will provide some food lists although, frankly, this is a damn simple diet.

In any case, in the last chapter I gave you a very simplified overview of human metabolism, which led into a discussion about what happens during starvation. This lets me bore you a little bit longer with a brief history lesson, which will act as a bridge to the diet itself.

A history lesson: From therapeutic starvation to the PSMF

As I mentioned in the previous chapter, therapeutic starvation for weight loss was great in terms of the weight/fat loss that it generated but had one huge problem associated with it: the loss of too much LBM. This sent researchers looking for a solution. Early studies tried giving small amounts of either carbohydrates or fats for energy. In the short term, at least, carbs did have some protein sparing effect. In the long-term, carbs were actually detrimental as they prevented the development and adaptation to ketosis. Fat didn't really have an effect either way except that it allowed ketosis to develop (because carbs weren't being eaten) so that the adaptations could take place.

Finally, someone got the bright idea to try just giving small amounts of proteins to see if this would allow all of the "benefits" of starvation without the large loss of body protein that was occurring. Voila, this worked and folks realized that the most protein-sparing nutrient of all is protein. Err, duh.

By providing dietary protein, the liver was now using dietary protein instead of body protein to make glucose, sparing the loss of LBM that had been occurring. This approach was called a protein sparing modified fast or PSMF.

Over the next few years, more studies were done examining a number of other variables, did adding carbs or fat to the dietary protein spare LBM, how much protein was needed to more or less completely eliminate the loss of body protein. Basically the goal was to find out what combination of nutrients would allow the least number of calories to be consumed while allowing the maximum rate of fat/weight loss and while sparing LBM losses.

After a good deal of experimentation, it was found that a protein intake of 1-1.5 grams of protein per kilogram of ideal body weight (IBW, this was used as a rough estimate of LBM although we'll be more technical about it) prevented the loss of body protein. For the non-metrically inclined, this works out to about 0.5-0.7 grams of protein per pound or so. So an individual with 150 pound of LBM would consume between 75 and 105 grams of protein and not much else beyond some vegetables, a lot of water, and a vitamin/mineral supplement. As described in the first chapter, this generated fat losses in the realm of ½ to 3/4 pounds per day and weight losses that were much higher due to water loss.

So that's it then, that's the diet?

So it took me all of these pages to basically tell you to eat nothing but a moderate amount of lean proteins with a few veggies, providing as few calories to your body as possible, so that you can lose weight and fat rapidly? Toss in a multivitamin/mineral and a lot of water and you're done, right? If that was the case, I could have written a pamphlet and been done with it. As is always the case with my books, there's more to do it.

What I'm going to propose in this booklet is actually a modified PSMF (no, I won't call it a mPSMF or something dumb like that). The goal, of course, is the same, to provide the body with all of the essential nutrients it needs while minimizing caloric intake as much as possible. This is to generate the greatest/most rapid weight/fat loss possible while sparing as much loss of LBM as possible. I'm simply addressing a few other issues that I feel are important for optimal results.

What modifications?

So let me talk a little bit about the modifications I'm going to make to the original PSMF. The first one is the addition of an essential fatty acid (EFA) source. Recall from Chapter 3 that there are two EFAs required by the body, referred to as omega-3 and omega-6 fatty acids.

For reasons that I really don't want to confuse or bore you with, we only need to worry about one of them in the short term: the omega-3 fatty acids. Now, the primary omega-3 fatty acid is alpha-linoleic acid or ALA (not to be confused with alpha-lipoic acid). As discussed in Chapter 3, this is found in some vegetable oils and food sources, but found in the greatest amount in flaxseed oil. ALA is broken down in the body, with extremely low efficiency, ultimately to the real players, the fish oils which are referred to as EPA and DHA (as before, trust me that you don't want to know what the letters stand for).

Now, odds are if you've watched TV or seen anything about diet in the supermarket checkout line, you've seen something about omega-3 fatty acids or fish oils. It's not an overstatement to say that they do nearly everything. They improve fat loss and insulin sensitivity, boost immune system function, decrease the risk of all manners of disease and have even been implicated in the prevention of diet-induced depression. If I hadn't read the research myself and saw a list of what omega-3s are purported to do, I'd think someone was conning me.

In addition to your daily protein requirement, an EFA source is required in my modified PSMF. Preformed fish oil capsules are best but not everybody likes taking a bunch of pills and they give some people nasty fish smelling burps (no joke); liquid fish oil products are also available. While concerns about purity and mercury contamination have been raised, invariably independent tests of commercial fish oil products find no problems. As mentioned previously, in the first edition of this book, I allowed for flaxseed oil as an alternative to fish oils but recent research has caused me to reverse this recommendation. Flaxseed oil is simply not an appropriate substitute for the fish oils.

Another modification that I'll be suggesting is in regards to protein intake. While the 1-1.5 g/kg ideal body weight (again, used as a proxy for LBM) is fine for very fat, inactive individuals, it isn't sufficient for leaner or more active individuals. I'm going to suggest that you set protein intake depending on activity level and fatness. I'll talk about how to determine your body fat level (or at least get a rough guesstimate) next chapter.

Another issue of course, is exercise. Some readers of this book are athletes who need to know how to train while on the PSMF for optimal results. Additionally, even sedentary individuals can benefit from adding certain types of exercise to the rapid fat loss plan and I'll give details about how to implement training with the diet.

Perhaps the biggest change I'm going to make to the original PSMF (in addition to the above modification) is the inclusion of deliberate breaks to the diet, periods when you will deliberately go off the diet to make it work better.

Of course, I'll also give you guidelines (as threatened in the foreword) for how long you should follow this type of diet before coming off of it. Once again, that depends on leanness level and, to a lesser degree in this case, activity.

These are the modifications that I'm going to discuss in detail in the next chapters (along with specifics of how to set up the diet of course). The overall scheme of the diet is summarized on the next page.

Summing up the rapid fat loss program

So let's sum up the modified PSMF. Each is discussed in more detail in upcoming chapters.

1. Protein intake set depending on body fat percentage and activity

2. Basically unlimited amount of vegetables (a few are off limits)

3. Either fish oil capsules or liquid fish oil for EFAs every day

4. A basic multivitamin/mineral supplement. One or two other key supplements.

5. Planned diet breaks depending on activity and body fat percentage

6. Length of PSMF to be set depending on body fat percentage and activity level

Estimating body fat percentage

In the last chapter, I made mention of how your starting body fat percentage will affect many aspects of how you set up this diet. If you recall from Chapter 1, body fat percentage refers to the amount of an individual's total body weight that is fat.

So imagine that we could wave a magic wand over you and say "Aha! You carry 22% body fat" or whatever the number might be. That means that, of your total body weight, 22% of it is comprised of fat. The rest, as per Chapter 1, is LBM.

Now, in addition to such things as overall health, how much body fat an individual is carrying affects numerous aspects of physiology. At least one of those is how their body will respond while dieting. Generally speaking, individuals who carry more body fat lose less LBM when they diet and they tend to have less problems with diet related metabolic slowdown (discussed in a later chapter). This has a number of implications for dieting, especially the rapid fat loss program.

Which means that it's time to talk about how to actually find out how much body fat you have. I should mention right now that, from this point forwards in the book, I'll be dividing dieters into different categories. Some of this division will be based upon starting body fat level; some of it will depend on activity (or lack thereof).

There are a number of methods of estimating body fat percentage (note the use of the word "estimating'; that's all it is, an estimate) ranging from low-tech to high-tech and from extremely accurate to horribly inaccurate. Which you use depends on your goals and what you have access to. I won't bore you listing all of the different methods; rather I'll focus on which ones I think are worth pursuing in this specific case.

Relatively lean individuals, athletes or bodybuilders, should either know what their body fat percentage is or have some reasonable method of estimating it. Although they have their own sets of problems, calipers would be my preferred method. If you know about calipers, I don't need to give you any more information; and if you don't, it won't do me any good to explain them. But I want to reiterate, if you're a relatively lean athlete, you will need a method of estimating body fat percentage outside of what I'm going to describe in this chapter.

Another possible method, although fraught with potential problems, are the bioelectrical impedance body fat scales (Tanita is a common brand). The problem is that these devices are drastically affected by hydration; a large glass of water or a big urination can alter the number. In general, I don't think they are that accurate but assuming you control for hydration, they can at least give you a starting point. I bring up the hydration issue because it will be affected greatly with this diet, making these types of scales nearly worthless.

Now, what about everybody else? Frankly, if you're not that lean and not currently very active, there's a fairly easy way to get a rough estimate of your body fat percentage and that is by using something called the Body Mass Index (BMI). BMI is supposed to be a measure of fatness but it's really not; what it does is relate height and weight with certain BMI ranges (supposedly) being associated with health or not. The problem with BMI is that it doesn't take body fat percentage into account.

That is, say we have two individuals who are 6 feet tall and weigh 200 pounds. But say one is an athlete and has 10% body fat (180 lbs LBM) and the other is not and has 30% body fat (140 lbs LBM). They will have the same BMI value but it's fairly clear (it should be anyhow) that they are not going to be in the same boat in terms of health risk, appearance or anything else. Basically, BMI makes no distinction between fat mass and LBM and since active individuals typically have more LBM (and hence less fat) at any given body weight, BMI is not accurate for them.

However, recent research has found that, with some limitations, BMI can be used to get a rough idea of body fat percentage. I want to make it abundantly clear that it's far from perfect and will provide, at best, an extremely rough estimate. However, since we're only looking for estimates in the first place, it's at least workable. But, again, keep in mind that the values you'll be deriving from Appendix 1 are only rough estimates, they are not holy writ and should not be considered as such.

As well, I must repeat: active individuals MUST find a different method (i.e. calipers or a Tanita scale or something) to estimate body fat; they cannot use the BMI method described in this chapter. Given that most active individuals probably have a rough idea of what their body fat percentage is in the first place, they are unlikely to need or use the method described in this chapter.

Please note that the online calculator will do all of the calculations in this (and subsequent chapters) automatically. Simply surf over to:

http://rapidfatlosshandbook.com/calculator.php

And enter the login/password combination that you received. I'd recommend reading the entire book before attempting to use the calculator however.

Determining BMI

BMI is not particularly difficult to calculate and the online calculator you received access to will do it for you when you're ready to set up the diet. As well, I've included charts to calculate BMI in Appendix 1. All you need to know is your height and scale weight. I've included both metric (weight in kilograms, height in meters) and Imperial (weight in pounds, height in feet and inches) values. Simply cross-reference your weight and height and find your BMI on the table. If you fall in-between values, just pick the middle value. Once again, we're not concerned with exacting accuracy, just a general idea.

Once you've determined your BMI, use table 2 in Appendix 1 to get a rough estimate of your body fat percentage. Again, the online calculator will do all of this for you automatically but I'll provide the calculations below if you want to do them yourself..

Putting the number to use

So now you have a rough estimate of your body fat percentage either based on some direct method (if you're active) or the BMI method (if you're not). There are two things I want you do now. The first is to determine how much of your total body weight is LBM. This is fairly simple. First you're going to multiply your current weight (either in pounds or kilograms) by your body fat percentage (divide the percentage by 100 so 30% becomes 0.30 for example) to determine how much of your total weight is fat.

$$\underline{\hspace{2cm}} * \underline{\hspace{1.5cm}} = \underline{\hspace{2cm}}$$
Weight   BF%   Total fat

Subtract the pounds of fat from your total weight, this is how much LBM you have.

$$\underline{\hspace{2cm}} - \underline{\hspace{1.5cm}} = \underline{\hspace{1.5cm}}$$
Total weight   Total fat   LBM

Your last task is to use Table 1 to determine what dieting category you are in (1, 2 or 3) based on your current body fat percentage. Please note that, to a degree, the separation between these categories are arbitrary, it would be more accurate to put them on a continuum. However, for ease of use, I have to make the divisions somewhere and this is where they fall. If you're right on the edge of a category, use the lower category. So a male who came in at 26% body fat should consider themselves in category 2, rather than category 3.

Table 1: Determining diet category based on body fat percentage

Category	Male BF%	Female BF%
1	15% and lower	24% and lower
2	16-25%	25-34%
3	26%+	35%+

As you lose fat, you may need to readjust which category you are in and adjust the various components of the diet accordingly. If you're already close to one of the cutoff points, you'll want to keep track of changes as that affects how you should set up the rest of the diet. If you're not, you can recheck every 4 weeks or so and recalculate BMI, body fat percentage, LBM and dieting category. This, of course, assumes that you're using the diet for more than the two weeks in the first place.

Exercise

Before we can get into finally setting up the diet, I need to talk a little about exercise, mainly because the type of exercise you choose to do while dieting will impact on the overall diet setup. That means defining the different types of exercise, talking about how exercise impacts on weight/fat loss, and finally having you decide what/if any exercise you'll be doing while you're on the crash diet.

Types of exercise

Ignoring the category of "none", there are three basic types of exercise that can be performed. The first is cardiovascular or aerobic exercise which generally refers to any activity that is performed more or less continuously for anywhere from 20 minutes up to several hours (in the case of highly trained athletes). I'd note that many also perform aerobic activity in smaller bouts throughout the day and this can be effective; performing 30 minutes per day in three ten-minute blocks throughout the day has been found to be similar to doing 30 minutes of continuous activity.

In any case, walking, running, cycling, swimming, step classes, the Stairmaster, etc. all of those fall under the heading of aerobic exercise. The goal of aerobic training is to burn calories and improve the health and fitness of the cardiovascular system (heart and lungs essentially) although there are many other adaptations that occur with this type of exercise.

In the past few years, a related form of training has become almost ridiculously popular (leading some to abandon regular cardio/aerobic training altogether), that method is interval training. Several studies have now shown that interval training can yield more effective fat loss than standard aerobic training although I don't think the conclusions are that cut and dry (for reasons I don't want to get into here).

Essentially a subcategory within aerobic training, interval/sprint training is performed with the same types of activities as aerobic training but entails working very hard for some short period of time (generally anywhere from 10 seconds to several minutes although 30-45 seconds would be more common than either extreme) and then taking it easy for some period of time (which depends on the length of the hard part).

So instead of performing 30 minutes of cycling at a moderate pace with regular aerobic training, with interval training you would warm-up for 5 minutes and then go nearly all out for 1-2 minutes at a time interspersed with 1-2 minutes of easy cycling (you might repeat that 5-10 times) and then cool-down. I'm really only mentioning interval training for completeness, it's neither appropriate or sustainable on the rapid fat loss plan.

Finally is resistance training which refers to any activity where the muscles are forced to work against a high resistance so that you are unable to continue the activity for more than a minute or so at a time. Most people think of this as lifting weights but working with rubber tubing, or many different home machines (such as Soloflex or Bowflex) also falls into this category. You could even fill milk jugs with water or sand and lift those. Or go to the park and lift rocks, or large pets, or small children.

For the most part, for reasons I'll discuss shortly, resistance training of some sort is the only type of exercise that you will need to perform on the rapid fat loss plan. There is some room for a small amount of low-intensity aerobic activity (although too much can be detrimental); intervals have no place on the diet.

Exercise and weight loss

You've probably heard, read or seen that you must exercise to lose weight/fat, or that exercising will drastically improve the amount or rate of weight or fat loss. It's important, once again, to make a distinction between weight and fat loss, as you'll see in a second.

People obviously can and do lose weight all the time without exercise (keeping the weight off is a separate issue I'll come back to below) so exercise certainly isn't required by any stretch. Whether or not programs that include exercise are optimal, better or more effective is an entirely different debate.

The question I want to address here is whether or not exercise has much of an effect on the rate of weight loss. For the most part, exercise has, at best, a small effect. Some studies find that it increases the total weight loss slightly while most find little to no effect. As I'll mention below, some studies find that exercise can actually reduce the total weight loss (note: as discussed previously in this book, not the same as fat loss).

Why? Why doesn't exercise improve the total rate of weight loss? The reason is one of simple mathematics and reality. Under most dieting conditions, unless a tremendous amount or a very high intensity of exercise can be done such that a very large amount of additional calories are burned, exercise simply fails to have much of an impact.

That is, unless you're capable of literally hours per day of exercise, sufficient to burn a ton of calories, the calorie burn from exercise will generally be quite small compared to the deficit created by food restriction. To burn 500-1000 calories per day with low intensity exercise would require hours of activity, to reduce food intake by that much may be much easier, at least in the short-term.

And the average overweight individual who is sedentary simply won't be able to burn enough calories with exercise to greatly impact on the overall deficit, at least not in the initial stages of their exercise program. Ironically, the only people who are able to burn a ton of calories with exercise are trained athletes, and they generally aren't the ones who need to lose a lot of fat in the first place.

Of course, over time, as people become fitter, both the amount and/or intensity of exercise can increase, increasing caloric expenditure. But this is not helpful for crash dieting. You can't improve fitness sufficiently in a two-week span to get much benefit from exercise.

This is even more the case on the rapid fat loss plan where the daily deficit is already pretty monstrous. That is, once you've generated a daily deficit in the realm of 1500-2000 calories/day (or higher in some cases), burning a few hundred more calories per day with exercise simply doesn't amount to much. Which isn't to say that exercise is useless but it's unrealistic to expect the addition of most exercise regimes to drastically increase the rate of weight loss.

Quite in fact, some studies suggest that there will be less *weight* loss if exercise is included during the diet but this is somewhat misleading. The reason is that, in beginner exercisers, exercise can cause an increase in LBM/muscle mass and this affects the amount of total *weight* that is lost. Less weight will be lost but only because LBM is being gained (or less LBM is being lost). I suspect that this is why some rapid weight loss centers actively recommend against exercise: they want to generate the greatest scale weight drops and that means avoiding anything that spares or increases LBM.

Of course, this is totally misleading, as I mentioned above. Maintaining (or even increasing) LBM on a diet, at the expense of fat loss shouldn't generally be construed as a bad thing. It's simply one of those places where focusing only on *weight* loss leads folks to bad conclusions and even worse recommendations. Which is part of why I spent all of Chapter 1 explaining the differences between weight and fat loss in the first place.

I should mention that, in the process of gaining weight, some proportion of that weight is LBM (some of which is muscle and some of which is simply connective tissue to support the extra weight) and most obesity experts accept some LBM loss as part of the weight loss. An LBM loss of 25-30% is usually considered acceptable in obese individuals since that represents the "extra" LBM they gained getting fat in the first place. But I digress.

What about fat loss?

Ok, so it looks like exercise, unless you are capable or willing to do hours of it per day, is unlikely to have a major effect on either the rate or total amount of weight loss. In some cases, exercise may actually decrease the total weight loss by increasing LBM. But that brings us back to the issue I brought up back in Chapter 1, the differentiation between weight loss and fat loss.

Because while exercise may not greatly affect the total amount of weight lost on a diet, it can affect the *composition* of what is lost, that is fat versus LBM. Depending on a host of variables, including the type and amount of exercise and the extent of the diet, some studies find that exercise (weight training more so than aerobic exercise) can alter the proportion of what is lost: more fat and less LBM are lost. In beginners at least, it's not uncommon to gain LBM while losing fat.

So even if total weight loss is the same (or slightly decreased), more fat is lost in the exercising group. Assuming your goal is fat loss and not *just* weight loss, exercise shouldn't generally be seen as detrimental. That is, even if your total weight loss ends up being decreased because you're exercising, a greater fat loss more than balances it out. Right?

As well, there are other potential benefits of exercising on a diet. Some studies indicate that exercise can help to prevent some of the metabolic slowdown that occurs with dieting. Please note that a great deal of research finds no such effect but it depends heavily on the type and amount of activity and how extreme the diet is (see next section). As well, some studies find that exercise helps dieters stick with their diet, adherence to the diet can be improved with the addition of exercise. At least within the context of the rapid fat loss program, this is probably one of the most important reasons to include it.

Can exercise hurt?

But can exercise be detrimental to weight or fat loss? In the case of a crash diet (or any extremely large deficit), the answer is a resounding yes. At least one study has found that the addition of a large amount of aerobic activity (roughly 6 hours per week) to a protein sparing modified fast *increased* the drop in metabolic rate that occurred. It didn't increase weight loss over the length of the study (4 weeks) either. Basically the caloric burn of the exercise led to an adaptive decrease in metabolic rate. Of course, the exercise also burned excess calories so the end result was the same.

As mentioned above, once you've generated a monster daily caloric deficit, burning a few hundred more calories through aerobic activity is unlikely to have much of an impact. I should mention that lighter dieters (usually women) often have to add some amount of aerobic activity along with a caloric deficit to achieve reasonable weekly fat loss although this generally shouldn't be the case on the rapid fat loss program.

Weight training hasn't been studied as extensively in this regards and I'm unaware of any studies on interval training in terms of how it might interact with the rapid fat loss program such as the one described in this booklet. Although I'll make more specific comments below, I'll say this upfront: unless it helps with adherence to the diet, I don't see much of a point in doing anything but the mildest aerobic activity on the crash diet. Thirty to forty minutes a few times per week (maybe daily) would be it.

Related to this, I've often seen what seems to be a thermodynamic impossibility, the combination of extremely large caloric deficits with an extremely large amount of activity (or a very high intensity of activity) often slows down or even stops fat loss completely. Yes, I know, it seems impossible but I've seen it happen enough times (including in myself) to know it happens.

Basically, if you want to create an extremely large caloric deficit through food restriction, you absolutely must not do too much activity (folks who have followed the diet in this

32

book have found this out the hard way, by ignoring my recommendations below and doing too much activity, they slowed their fat and weight loss). If you want to do a lot of activity, you cannot cut calories too severely. Again, I know this doesn't make much sense and I'm still trying to pin down the mechanisms of why this happens. But the simple fact is that it does and if you want to avoid problems, you must follow the recommendations I'm going to give below in terms of how much exercise you can or should do.

Frankly, weight training a maximum of 2-3 times per week is going to be the best form of exercise on the rapid fat loss plan. A small amount of low intensity aerobic activity (I mean brisk walking), if it helps with diet adherence is acceptable as well. Intervals are inappropriate and should not be done, they simply can't be recovered from on so few calories, especially not if proper weight training is being performed. I'll give more specific recommendations below.

Why weight training? Well, outside of the reasons discussed above, the reason is that we want to lose predominantly body fat. Maintaining (for experienced exercisers) or increasing (for beginners) LBM on the rapid fat loss plan is the primary goal and nothing will accomplish that more effectively than weight training. The massive daily caloric deficit will take care of the fat loss, more calorie burning activity simply isn't necessary or useful; as discussed above, done in excess it can be detrimental.

Preventing weight regain

As a final comment, I want to mention that a rather large amount of research suggests that exercise may play its major role in preventing weight regain after a diet is over. Studies routinely show that individuals who get involved in regular exercise are more likely to maintain the weight/fat loss than those who don't.

This would be one reason for folks who are not on an exercise program to start at least something (even if it's only doing light weight training at home coupled with some brisk walking) during the rapid fat loss plan, you'll be in a position to get into a more formalized exercise program once you come off the diet (discussed in more detail in Chapters 11-15). If you choose not to begin an exercise program while on the rapid fat loss plan, you should give some consideration to starting one once it's over.

That assumes, of course, that you want to maintain the weight/fat you lost. Note that studies of successful dieters (individuals who have lost weight and kept it off long-term) find involvement in a regular exercise program as one of several common behavior patterns.

I'll mention up front that it appears to take quite a bit of activity, along the lines of 2500 calories burned per week through exercise to maintain the weight loss. That works out to a solid 1.5 hours of moderate intensity activity or about an hour of hard activity pretty much daily. Smaller amounts of exercise have progressively smaller effects.

The basics of resistance training

As discussed above, properly performed weight training is going to be the most important type of activity that you can perform on the rapid fat loss plan. As also mentioned above, resistance training can encompass a tremendous number of different activities from formal weight lifting to machine circuits to rubber tubing to even bodyweight exercises (for folks who work out at home). When you bought this book, you received an additional book showing a basic home bodyweight based exercise program that you can use.

But before getting into specifics, I want to talk a little more generally about the topic of resistance training. First I want to explain some terms for people who are wholly unfamiliar with resistance training, those appear in the box below. If you are already on an established weight-training program, you can skip down a bit to the next section which talks about specifics.

Basic Weight Training Terminology

Repetition (rep): the raising and lowering of the resistance once is referred to as one rep (or repetition).

Set: A set is a series of repetitions. So if you lifted a weight 8 times and then stopped, you would have done one set of 8 repetitions.

Rest interval (RI): Between sets of the same exercise, you typically rest (doing nothing), and this rest may last anywhere from 15-30 seconds up to several minutes, depending on the specifics of the training program.

Frequency: This is simply how often you exercise, typically individuals will perform resistance training anywhere from two to seven days per week (some very advanced or simply very obsessed athletes will lift more than once per day). Within the context of the rapid fat loss plan, two to three days per week of resistance training is more than enough.

Muscle group: This simply refers to the muscle or muscles that are targeted by a given exercise. A biceps curl may work only the biceps (the muscle on the front of the arms) while a squat may work the glutes, hamstrings and quadriceps (muscles of the lower body)

Very simplistically, resistance training can be divided into two different "types" when it comes to training for maximum fat loss.

The stock-standard approach to resistance training is to generally use fairly heavy weights for anywhere from 5-12 repetitions per set and for multiple sets (typically more than one exercise per muscle group is done as well). I want to make it clear that, unless you're being coached, low repetitions are inappropriate for beginners. Keeping the repetitions at 8 or higher is generally safer. In any case, the idea behind this type of training while dieting is that it works the most effectively for maintaining LBM. One of the biggest mistakes that experienced trainers can do when they diet is to lower the intensity of their resistance training (by increasing the number of repetitions) too much; this causes LBM loss.

A popular approach recently is to use high repetitions (generally 12-15 but sometimes even higher), short-rest periods, and multiple sets. I described this in my Ultimate Diet 2.0 as depletion training; others call it by different names. But the basic goal is the same. This type of resistance training tends to burn more calories, deplete glycogen (carbohydrate stored in the muscle; this is beneficial as it increases fat burning), generates a nice hormonal response in terms of fat mobilization and may create a larger caloric burn after the exercise is done. This is the most appropriate type of resistance training for beginners from both a safety and effectiveness standpoint. More advanced trainees will often perform this type of training in addition to the heavier work described above.

With that background given, I now want to outline some sample exercise routines both for those not already on an exercise program (discussed first) and then for those who have already been training for a while but who are using the rapid fat loss program.

For beginners not already on an exercise program

I can't assume that everybody reading this book is already on an exercise program. Quite in fact, it's probably safe to assume that many, if not most, are not. Given the nature of the rapid fat loss program, it's therefore very important that folks know how to safely and effectively begin an exercise program.

I do want to mention that for individuals in Category 3, maintenance of LBM while dieting, especially when protein intake is sufficient, usually isn't a huge problem. The more body fat someone is carrying, the less LBM they will lose under any circumstances. So if you simply can't or won't begin an exercise program while on the rapid fat loss program, that's probably fine in the short-term. As you'll learn in later chapters, exercise may play its most important role in keeping the weight and fat off when the diet is ended.

But assuming that you're interested in beginning a basic exercise program, which of course I highly recommend, read on. If not, you can go to the next chapter which explains how to set up the diet itself.

Perhaps the single most important piece of advice I can give to beginners regarding starting an exercise program is to start slowly and build up gradually. If there's a single way to ensure that you won't stick with an exercise program, it's to start with far too much and either get so sore or so overwhelmed that you don't make it past the first day.

Trust me when I say that this is all too common an occurrence: someone decides to start exercising, overdoes it the first day, can't walk for the next week and that's the beginning and end of the program. Better to start more slowly and build up more gradually. That way, by the time you're actually doing a lot of exercise (or training very intensely), the increase has been so gradual that you never really felt overwhelmed by the program.

One nice thing about being completely new to exercise is that it doesn't take very much to generate a response in terms of getting stronger or gaining or maintaining LBM. In the section above I defined sets; here I only want to mention that numerous studies find that, for beginners, a single set gives essentially identical results to doing more than one set. This isn't to say that increasing the number of sets done over time can't be useful or isn't a good idea, only that, in the beginning, there's little to no need to do more than that.

For that reason, in the sample exercise programs below, I strongly suggest that beginners perform only a single set to begin with. I'll talk about how to progress the training program (if desired) as well.

Another issue for beginners is lifting speed; this refers to how quickly (or slowly) the reps are done. For beginners, there's really little to discuss. For both safety reasons and from the standpoint of learning the exercises, I recommend that beginners use fairly slow and controlled movement speeds. Lifting the weight in two seconds and lowering it in two seconds would be an appropriate speed. This would make each repetition last four seconds.

Finally is the issue of breathing. Generally speaking, when lifting any type of resistance, beginners are best served by exhaling as they lift the weight and inhaling as they lower it. However, far more importantly is that people make sure to breathe in the first place; I've often seen beginners hold their breath and end up gasping for air midway through a set. It's more important *that* you breathe than *how* you breathe.

A beginning weight trainer should be performing the most basic of routines. At most one exercise per bodypart should be done and the whole body should be worked at each workout with higher repetitions (12-15) and lighter weights.

As mentioned above, this accomplishes a number of important goals: it burns calories, will decrease the carbohydrate stored in muscle (which increases how much fat the body burns at rest) and tends to be safer and more effective in the beginning stages of training.

If you belong to a gym, this type of routine can be done easily and quickly using machines or free weights (barbells or dumbbells). If you don't belong to a gym, the accompanying e-book contains some basic exercises that can be done at home using the minimum amount of equipment. The workout itself would be done a maximum of two to three times per week (three is the absolute maximum) on nonconsecutive days. If you decided to exercise twice per week, you would want to spread the days out across the week. Monday and Thursday or Monday and Friday or some similar spacing (e.g. Tuesday/Friday) would be ideal. If you exercise three times per week, you would exercise Monday/Wednesday/Friday or Tuesday/Thursday/Saturday.

In the box on the next page, I've included two sample routines for beginning exercisers; one is a basic gym routine if you have access, the other is a basic home routine that can be done. If you need or want more details than that, you can go purchase one of the dozens of beginning weight training books on the market. This will get you started.

Beginner Exercise Routines

Gym routine	Sets	Reps	RI	Home Routine	Sets	Reps	RI
Leg press	1-3	12-15	1'	Squat or lunge	1-3	12-15	1'
Leg curl*	1-3	12-15	1'	Glute bridge*	1-3	12-15	1'
Chest press	1-3	12-15	1'	Push-up	1-3	12-15	1'
Rowing	1-3	12-15	1'	1-arm row	1-3	12-15	1'
Lateral raise*	1-2	12-15	1'	Lateral raise*	1-2	12-15	1'
Biceps curl*	1-2	12-15	1'	Biceps curl*	1-2	12-15	1'
Triceps pushdown*	1-2	12-15	1'	Chair dips*	1-2	12-15	1'
Crunch	1-3	12-15	1'	Crunch	1-3	12-15	1'
Back extension	1-3	12-15	1'	Bird dogs	1-3	12-15	1'

* Indicates optional exercises, this is described in more detail in the text

A few notes about the above routines:

Each of the exercises listed above is demonstrated in the book that you received when you purchased this manual. For the exercises that require them, the home exercise manual demonstrates each using milk jugs. Dumbbells or home exercise tubing can also be used and, in the long-term, will give more flexibility and exercise options.

Although sets are listed as 1-3, I highly recommend that beginners start with only one set of each exercise on their first day. As mentioned above, an excellent way to completely derail an exercise program is to start with too much too soon. If the first day is extremely easy, you can always add a second set during your second workout. If it's still challenging, stick with the single set.

Although the repetitions are listed as 12-15, not everyone will get to 15 repetitions, especially on bodyweight exercises (weight machines at the gym can always be set very light) initially. I recommend that you stick with the exercise until you can get 15 repetitions fairly comfortably before considering adding a second set. Once you can do 2 sets of 15 easily, you can consider adding a third set. Or you can add weight instead of adding sets as discussed two paragraphs below on progression.

RI stands for rest interval, which I have set at one minute across the board. If you're only doing one set of each exercise, this means that you would rest one minute between exercises. If you are doing multiple sets of an exercise, you should rest one minute between sets. So say you are doing 3 sets of 12-15 leg presses. You do your first set of 15, rest a minute, do a second set of 15, rest a minute, do a third set, rest a minute, then move on to your next exercise.

One factor I haven't talked about yet is progression. To get stronger (or build bigger muscles), you have to overload them by making them work harder. For beginners, this usually means adding more weight to the exercise to make it more difficult. So once you can do 15 repetitions easily with say, 10 pounds, you would move to 12 or 15 pounds. This might bring you back down to 12 repetitions, then you'd build back up to 15 repetitions, once that got easy, you'd add weight again. Beginners can generally use this type of approach for quite some time before needing anything more complicated.

For the home exercise routine, progression can be a bit more difficult. I've included some more advanced movements in the home exercise manual that you got with this book but eventually even those may become too easy. Adding weight by using small dumbbells, plates (both of which can usually be purchased fairly inexpensively at various sporting goods stores, or found used) can be used.

Exercises marked with a * should be considered optional. They can be performed if you have energy, time or inclination but are not required. The goal of this routine is to hit the greatest amount of muscle mass with the least number of exercises. If you only performed the main exercises, you would have covered your bases.

So that's the nuts and bolts of a basic resistance training program. Now I want to make a few comments about aerobic activity. As discussed above, the addition of too much cardio to an extreme diet like this one can cause more problems than it solves, causing a greater reduction in metabolic rate (without increasing weight loss) than would otherwise occur.

Even so, a small amount of aerobic/cardiovascular type of exercise can be performed and this often helps with diet adherence. Many people tend to link exercising with eating "better", doing a small amount of aerobic activity often helps with the diet in this fashion.

Beginners should start with a minimum of 20 minutes three times per week at a fairly low intensity. Walking works just fine although other types of activity can also be done. If you're doing your weight training program at a gym, you can do your cardio afterwards. If you're exercising at home (or not doing resistance training at all), brisk walking can be done (weather allowing) outdoors any time. If beginners want to increase the amount of time they do aerobic activity, this can be done gradually. But no more than perhaps 30' per day should be performed for the reasons discussed above. Once the diet is over and calories are increased, more activity (or more intense activity) can be pursued in order to help with weight maintenance.

As far as intervals are concerned, exercisers shouldn't do intervals until they've got a solid 8-12 weeks of basic beginner training under their belt in the first place. They aren't appropriate during the rapid fat loss program anyhow. As with increasing amounts (or intensity) of aerobic activity discussed in the paragraph above, intervals could be incorporated once calories have been increased (see the later chapters of this book) to help with weight maintenance.

Guidelines for exercise: Athletes and those already exercising

Having discussed those not already on an exercise program, I now want to talk about individuals using the rapid fat loss program who are already on an established exercise program. These are likely to be athletes, bodybuilders or simply obsessed exercisers/dieters who are using the rapid fat loss program to reduce their body fat. In general, I'd expect them to be Category 1 or 2 dieters although this certainly isn't always going to be the case (many super-heavyweight powerlifters or Olympic lifters carry a good bit of body fat but may still need to reduce body fat rapidly).

Clearly, you will want to keep up your training program on the rapid fat loss plan, the question then becomes one of how best to do it. Essentially, you should keep up your training program but the total volume and frequency of your training should be cut way back; you simply won't have the recovery capacity on so few calories.

Studies routinely show that both volume (number of sets, amount of aerobic training done) and frequency (days/week) can be cut back significantly (by up to 2/3rds) as long as intensity (e.g. weight on the bar) is maintained. Given those parameters, performance can be maintained for many weeks. If you're as overtrained as most athletes, cutting back on your training during a crash diet will act as a mini-taper, you might even show some improvement. But don't hold your breath for this to occur.

In general, I'd say cut your weight training back to twice/week maximum doing a full body workout at each session. Two to three heavy sets of 6-8 repetitions are more than sufficient in the short-term to maintain LBM and strength. The Category 1 rapid fat loss dieters who have had the most success with the diet are the one that have cut back their training volume to these low levels.

Yes, I know that full body workouts are out of vogue and dieting bodybuilders are almost pathological in their desire to increase both the frequency and volume of training when they are contest dieting but this is a mistake, more so during a crash diet. Trust me on this: cut your training back during this diet. You are likely to get into real problems if you try to train too frequently or too much on too few calories: don't say you weren't warned.

A sample routine appears in the box below.

Sample Full Body Exercise Routine			
Exercise	Sets	Reps	RI
Squat or leg press	2-3	6-8	2-3'
RDL or leg curl	1-2	6-8	2-3'
Bench press or Incline DB press	2-3	6-8	2-3'
Rowing or chins	2-3	6-8	2-3'
Lateral raise	1-2	8-10	1-2'
Biceps	1-2	8-10	1-2'
Triceps	1-2	8-10	1-2'
Weighted crunch	1-2	6-8	1-2'
Back extension	1-2	6-8	1-2'

Of course you could also perform two slightly different workouts on each of your two workout days. So do squat, bench press, row (and some accessory stuff) on Day 1 and Deadlifts (or leg press), incline bench, chins (and some accessory stuff) on Day 2. You'll hit everything, maintain your LBM and strength and let the diet take care of the fat loss.

If you're desperate to work out more frequently than twice weekly, I'd suggest using an Upper/Lower split routine alternated on a Monday/Wednesday/Friday (or Tuesday/Thursday/Saturday) schedule but with extremely reduced volume. So your training over two weeks would look like this, with each workout being performed three times in two weeks.

Monday: Upper	Monday: Lower
Wednesday: Lower	Wednesday: Upper
Friday: Upper	Friday: Lower

Your workout shouldn't take long, maybe forty minutes in and out the door. A sample workout appears in the box below. Again, the goal is to do the least amount of work that will maintain strength and LBM. The below may not seem like much work but, on the low calories of the rapid fat loss program, it's plenty.

Sample Upper/Lower Split

Upper body workout				Lower body workout			
Exercise	Sets	Reps	RI	Exercise	Sets	Reps	RI
Bench press or Incline DB press	2-3	6-8	2-3'	Squat or Leg press	2-3	6-8	2-3'
Row or chin	2-3	6-8	2-3'	RDL	2-3	6-8	2-3'
Lateral raise	1-2	8-10	1-2'	Calf raise	2-3	6-8	2-3'
Biceps	1-2	8-10	1-2'	Weighted crunch	2-3	6-8	2-3'
Triceps	1-2	8-10	1-2'	Back extension	2-3	6-8	2-3'

Finally, one option to consider (for Category 1 dieters especially) is to begin the short diet cycle with some high rep work (3-6 sets of 12-15 reps) at the very start of the diet to deplete muscle glycogen and enhance fat oxidation (see my Ultimate Diet 2.0 for more information on how to implement this). The remainder of the workouts over the length of the diet would be short, heavy, full body workouts as described above. After the depletion work at the beginning of the cycle, a short full body workout would be done every 3-4 days afterwards. Again, this may not seem like much work but is more than enough.

I want to add that the low blood glucose that typically occurs on a low-carb diet can really sap training intensity, especially in the weight room. This is probably a central effect; the brain simply isn't sending neural signals to the muscles as well when blood glucose is low. Consuming 5 grams of carbohydrate (I'll mention this again in another chapter) about 10 minutes before you train can help a lot with your ability to maintain intensity, by increasing blood glucose back to the normal range.

Conceivably, dieters could even increase this to 15-30 grams of carbs taken during the workout (this only adds 60-120 calories to your diet) as well. If you want to save some of your protein intake and consume it around training (maybe 15 grams of whey immediately before and/or after the workout), this will help to support protein synthesis and limit LBM losses as well. This will decrease how much food you are able to consume for the remainder of the day.

And what about cardio? Well, as above, too much cardio when added to a crash diet such as this one can cause more problems than it solves. At the same time, the leaner people get (12-15% or lower for men, 21-24% or lower for women) some cardio certainly appears to help with fat loss. This is especially true for women and losing lower body fat than it is for men (many male bodybuilders can get ripped simply with lifting and diet).

Again, don't go crazy with it. Twenty minutes of low intensity cardio after you lift is plenty. Another couple of days of perhaps thirty to forty minutes (only if you have very good recovery) would be more than sufficient. More isn't better unless you want to over-train, lose LBM and actually slow down your fat loss results.

I should address non-bodybuilding athletes who are using the rapid fat loss program to drop weight and fat rapidly (to make a weight class or what have you). Due to the massive caloric deficit, you should reduce training as much as possible. Metabolic work should be scaled way back (preferably to only low intensity work) and the above recommendations for weight work still holds. Technical work should be doable but don't be shocked if you run out of gas pretty quickly. The same recommendations for taking a small amount of pre-workout or during-workout carbs would apply in these situations. Just remember that the rapid fat loss plan is short-term only.

As mentioned above, if you're as overtrained as most athletes are, odds are a reduction in training volume and frequency might do you some good. If you feel that you absolutely must maintain an extremely high level of training, you will have to choose another dietary approach, the rapid fat loss program simply won't work. In the future, try to keep your body fat under control so that you're never in the situation of having to crash diet in the first place.

The possibility of including interval training on the rapid fat loss plan is probably one of the most common questions I get, especially with the current fascination that the fitness world has with them; this was not helped by the fact that I allowed that they might be possible in the First Edition of this book. To simplify both my life and yours, I'm taking a stronger stance on intervals this time. Don't do them. You won't be able to recover from them and you won't be able to do them well in the first place. If you feel that your program simply must include interval training, pick a different diet. I hope that's clear enough.

42

Setting up the diet

And finally it's time to actually set up the daily diet. In this chapter, you're going to use the diet category you're in (1,2, or 3 from the last chapter) along with your LBM and the type of exercise you're doing (or not doing) to determine your daily protein intake for the rapid fat loss program. Once again, the online calculator will do all of the steps described in this chapter automatically but each step is described below as well.

http://rapidfatlosshandbook.com/calculator.php

I talked about exercise in the last chapter and, by this point you should know what, if anything, you will be doing. In this chapter, you're going to put all of that information to use to set up your daily diet.

In actuality, it's quite simple; just use Table 1 below. In the far left column are the different diet categories; on the top is a listing of activity, either no activity, aerobic activity only, or weight training (this would include weight training and aerobics). Just find your category on the left and cross-reference it with the activity on the top and that's your daily protein intake per pound of LBM.

Table 1: Daily protein intake based on activity and diet category

Category	Inactive	Aerobic	Weight training
1	1.25	1.5	2.0
2	0.9	1.1	1.25
3	0.8	0.9	1.0

Note: all values are grams protein per pound of LBM

Pretty simple, really. Now, one last step and I swear you're done with math (well, until the last chapters anyhow). Now you have to multiply your LBM in pounds by the number from Table 1, that's your daily protein intake. Metric readers should multiply their weight in kg by 2.2 to get pounds and then multiply by protein intake in gram per pound to get total grams of protein per day. The calculation is shown in the box below.

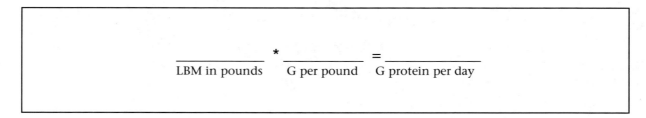

So if you have 150 pounds of LBM and are in Category 1 and doing weight training, you will need 150 * 2 = 300 grams of protein per day. An individual with 100 pounds LBM in Category 2 doing light aerobic activity would need 100 * 1.1 = 110 grams of protein per day. Finally, a Category 3 dieter with 110 pounds of LBM who is only doing light aerobic activity would need 110 * 0.8 = 88 grams of protein per day. I'll talk about what to eat and how to divide it up momentarily.

What do I eat?

So you're wondering what to eat each day, maybe hoping I'll fill the rest of this booklet with hundreds of pages of interesting recipes. Unfortunately, I'm not that kind of diet book author and this isn't that kind of diet book. Nor is this a diet that lends itself to such an approach in the first place. You'll find, as you read through the next sections that your food options are fairly limited and any individual meal will end up being extremely simple. Which isn't to say that I won't give you some guidelines, I simply want to make the point that this is not an exciting or interesting diet; it's supposed to be effective, not fun.

I will, however, give you some guidance on what to eat. It should be pretty clear that you're going to be limited to protein sources that are low in both fat and carbohydrates. Some rapid fat loss dieters have taken this to an extreme, attempting to choose foods that contain zero grams of either fat or carbohydrates. They figure that if the diet says protein only, that's what it means.

While this may appeal to a certain level of obsessive compulsiveness among the sorts of people who read my books, for the majority, I think it can be problematic since it tends to desperately limit the number of foods that can be eaten. By allowing a small amount of carbohydrate or fat grams per serving of protein, many more foods can be eaten, allowing for more flexibility and increasing adherence down the road.

For example, low-fat cottage cheese typically contains about four grams of carbohydrates and 2.5grams of fat per serving along with 13 grams of protein (note: these numbers can vary significantly and you'll have to read the label to be sure). One serving of that at a given meal would certainly be allowed (the rest of the meal would have to be essentially fat and carbohydrate free protein sources). Similarly, extremely lean ground beef often has as little as 4 grams of fat per 3 oz. serving, along with 21-24 grams of protein or so. That would also be acceptable. In contrast, a glass of milk (or cup of yogurt) containing 14 grams of carbohydrate per serving with only 8 grams of protein would be unacceptable; it has too many carbohydrates with too little protein.

But I need to put in a warning here: it's easy to go from a "few" grams of carbohydrates or fat per serving of protein to a "lot" of grams of either and suddenly you're back to eating exactly how you ate before. That defeats the purpose of the diet.

Recall from an earlier chapter that the goal of the diet is to provide the essential nutrients (protein, EFAs, nutrients found in vegetables) while limiting everything else. The more tagalong carbohydrate and fats that you add, the further away from the principle of the rapid fat loss diet that you get. So it's always a compromise. Allowing a bit more food flexibility can help adherence (as well as preparing you better for when the diet is ended) but don't get so flexible that you end up limiting your fat losses or ruin the diet.

In any case, I strongly suggest that you get into the habit of reading labels, you'd be surprised at how many hidden grams of carbs and fat turn up in what you'd think are pure protein sources. This isn't as limiting as it might seem and some of the best food sources appear in the list below. Again note that most protein sources can contain a gram or two of fat or carbs without it being any big deal within the big scheme of this diet.

Low-fat and low-carbohydrate protein sources

Skinless chicken or turkey breast: If you buy commercially prepared products, you need to watch out for various flavorings and such that often contain a lot of hidden carbohydrates

Low-fat fish: tuna, cod, halibut, flounder, lobster, crab

Extremely lean red meat: As noted above, this can often be found with as little as 4 grams of fat per serving which is an acceptable amount.

Fat free cheese: This can be added to other protein sources (such as egg whites or to top a lean hamburger) to bump up the protein content without adding many extra carbohydrate or fat grams.

Low- fat cottage cheese: as mentioned above, this is acceptable in moderation (no more than one serving at any given meal) as it contains some fat and carbohydrates along with the protein

Egg whites

Beef jerky: Can contain quite a few carbs depending on the flavoring, read the label.

Protein powder: See comments below

45

Admittedly it's not a huge list of foods but this is also a short-term diet. Additionally, making the above foods part of your habitual diet will be good for maintenance eating when the diet is over (discussed in detail in Chapters 11-15). As well, you should be able to keep yourself interested by mixing and matching.

For example, melt some fat free cheese on top of lean ground beef, throw on some lettuce, tomatoes and mustard and make a cheeseburger. Or make an omelet out of egg whites and the same fat free cheese (throw in some veggies to plump it up), many dieters will make a dessert of sorts out of cottage cheese with some chocolate protein powder and some Splenda, you get the idea.

Ok, let's talk about dairy. I highly recommend you get one to three servings of dairy in your daily meal plan. There are at least two reasons for this. The first is that calcium is turning out to have important benefits in terms of fat loss and some studies suggest that dairy calcium works better than other forms: high dairy calcium fat loss diets cause greater fat loss than either low-calcium or nondairy calcium diets. Calcium is also an important nutrient for overall bone health anyhow and the calcium from dairy is absorbed the best (I'll talk about calcium supplements below).

The second is of more relevance for athletes and lean individuals but one of the proteins in dairy (casein) has been shown to spare LBM loss. Frankly, this isn't a huge deal for Category 2 and 3 dieters but is extremely important for Category 1 dieters. An additional benefit of dairy protein is that milk protein (casein) digests very slowly; it tends to sit in the stomach a long time. This helps to increase fullness for longer after a meal.

So what about protein powders which are a staple of athletes and bodybuilders (and sometimes used by other dieters), what is their place on this diet? Frankly, I don't think protein powders should make up the bulk of the daily diet (on this or any other diet) although they can be used sparingly. If you are an obsessed weight trainer, bodybuilder or athlete and just must use a protein powder, use whey protein right around your workouts as I mentioned in the last chapter.

I will be the first to admit that just measuring out powders makes it extremely easy to control food intake. This is probably why many previous approaches to the PSMF have relied on liquid nutrition and shakes. Quite in fact, I considered designing a meal replacement powder to go along with this diet and would probably make a tremendously greater amount of money doing so. Unfortunately, I think the cons of using powdered/liquid nutrition far outweigh that benefit. I suppose if someone rolled a truckload of money to my door, I'd consider it.

The problem in my mind is that, while this approach to dieting generates amazing weight/fat loss in the short term, it does nothing to teach or retrain overall eating habits in the longer term. I'll talk about this more in the chapters on how to end this diet but recall that one use of the rapid fat loss plan is to jump start a normal diet, I'll also talk about how to maintain the weight loss (assuming such is your goal) in those chapters.

But doing that means relearning an overall better way of eating and that means eating real food during the diet. Structuring the crash diet around such liquid products is probably easier in the short run but I feel that it will ultimately be limiting in the long run. I'd rather see rapid fat loss dieters get into the habit of making good whole food choices for when they come off the diet. In any case, back to protein powders.

One of the cons is that protein powders tend to leave people hungry as they digest fairly rapidly unless combined with a soluble fiber (think guar gum or psyllium husks). One exception is the protein I mentioned above, casein. Due to its chemical structure, casein forms a "clot" in the stomach, and digests extremely slowly. However, casein protein by itself tends to taste a bit chalky, mix poorly and isn't that readily available. But another protein, called milk protein isolate (or MPI) is available, and contains about 80% casein (with 20% whey). Many Category 1 rapid fat loss dieters have used MPI for part of their protein intake and find that it keeps them full for absolutely hours.

For folks who have never used protein powder before, I would still recommend relying primarily on whole foods during the rapid fat loss diet. As mentioned above, I think this is better for a lot of reasons. If you want to obtain some MPI to try out there are numerous places online to obtain it, either in bulk or as a commercial product. I'd recommend you start with a small quantity at first, in case you don't like the stuff. You can always order more if you do like it. Or, just stick with food.

The rest of the diet: Vegetables, EFAs, water and supplements

Compared to dealing with protein intake, which is mainly an issue of determining how much you need (using the equation above) and which foods fit that goal, the rest of the diet is fairly simple. The three components I want to talk about now are vegetables, the essential fatty acids (EFAs), water intake and any supplements that may be useful or necessary (one specific supplement will get discussed in its own separate chapter).

Be honest with yourself for a second, you know you don't eat enough vegetables. You also know that they are good for you and that your grandmother was right all along about them. Why are vegetables important? Well, among other things, they are a primary source of vitamins and minerals in the diet, in addition to containing a class of nutrients called phytonutrients (or phytochemicals) that are turning out to have a number of health benefits. While I still recommend a basic one-per-day multivitamin on this (or any) diet, consuming lots of vegetables will go a long way to ensure good nutrient intake.

The fiber content of vegetables also helps with regularity (in terms of bowel movements) in addition to helping with fullness (the sheer volume of vegetables helps to fill the stomach). Since they are crunchy, they give the diet texture; they also tend to take a while to eat. This is important, as there is a delay between when you eat and when your brain realizes that you're full. I'll discuss this more in a later chapter.

Vegetables can also provide snacks in between meals to help keep hunger at bay. Since you will need extra sodium anyhow (see below), a cucumber or bag of celery and a saltshaker can help with munchies for snacking.

So which vegetables? As mentioned in an earlier chapter, some vegetables actually contain quite a bit of carbohydrate; these are often referred to as "starchy vegetables". Foods such as peas, carrots, corn, potatoes (normal and sweet) and beets are a few examples, there are probably others but these are the most commonly eaten ones. These foods are off-limits on the rapid fat loss plan. Yes, fine, if you want a little bit of sliced carrot for your salad, that's acceptable. Don't think you can eat a half a potato because it's a vegetable; it has too many carbohydrates

The other "class" of vegetables is commonly referred to as fibrous vegetables; a partial list appears below. In general, fibrous vegetables have very few digestible carbohydrates, although they do have some. For example, 3 oz (85 grams) of broccoli can contain 2 grams of digestible carbohydrate along, with 2 grams of fiber and 3 grams of protein; 3 oz is not very much broccoli. In contrast, many types of lettuce are essentially calorie free.

Fibrous Vegetables				
Asparagus	Green beans	Broccoli	Brussel sprouts	Cabbage
Cauliflower	Celery	Cucumbers	Eggplant	Lettuce
Mushrooms	Green peppers	Red peppers	Spinach	Zucchini

Clearly this isn't a comprehensive list as there are tons more vegetables available than this. If you're unsure if a given food is acceptable or not, go look it up. The following website has an extremely comprehensive database of foods. You simply enter the food you want, choose from the list of possibilities it gives you and then enter the amount (e.g. one small tomato).

http://www.calorieking.com

In the first edition of this book, I said that rapid fat loss dieters could eat essentially unlimited amounts of fibrous vegetables and I want to amend that slightly here by giving readers a quick reality check. On the one hand, it's unlikely that most are going to consume such a massive amount of fibrous vegetables that they will contribute a huge number of calories. But it can certainly happen. At the same time, I don't want to put some sort of arbitrary intake value or number since this only adds an unneeded level of complexity to what should otherwise be a fairly simple diet. A couple of examples should help to make my point.

Consider a light female who only be consuming 400-500 calories per day on the rapid fat loss plan. If she went nuts with fibrous vegetables, eating several cups of the above at each of her four meals, she might easily add over 200 calories to her diet; that would represent nearly 50% of her daily intake, cutting her daily deficit (and fat loss) considerably. Contrast this to a large male who might be consuming 800-1000 calories (or more), that same vegetable intake might be absolutely fine.

My point is not that you should automatically limit your vegetable intake; I strongly suggest you consume some at each meal to keep you full, etc. At the same time, don't abuse vegetables to the point that you derail the diet and reduce (or eliminate your supposed deficit).

A potential problem is what to put on top of your vegetables since most salad dressings and toppings contain either sugar or fat. Lemon juice with spices is always an easy option and some of the vinegar-based dressings (vinaigrettes) are essentially calorie free. I've listed some "free foods" at the end of the chapter which can be mixed and matched to spice up your meals.

In a previous chapter, I talked about the essential fatty acids (EFAs) but I really want to drive home the need to supply the omega-3's on the rapid fat loss plan. Although there is a second EFA, the omega-6 fatty acid, the body actually has a rather large store of it and it's altogether too common in the modern food supply. For a short-term diet like the rapid fat loss plan, worrying about omega-6 intake is unnecessary. So how do you get your omega-3's?

Several years ago, the popular recommendation was to consume flaxseed oil (some actually ate ground up flax seeds themselves) as this contains one of the "parent" omega-3 fats (called alpha-linoleic acid or ALA); I even allowed for this in the first edition of this book. Unfortunately, the body is extremely inefficient at converting ALA to the important compounds which are EPA and DHA (again, you don't need to or want to know what these letters stand for). For that reason, I prefer that dieters take pre-formed fish oils capsules or use liquid fish oil (Carlson's is a common brand). This is the only truly effective way to raise the body's levels of EPA and DHA.

How much EFA per day? Recent research has found that the body will saturate tissue levels of the EPA and DHA at an intake of roughly 1.8 grams EPA and 1.2 grams of DHA. This works out to 10 standard one-gram fish oil capsules. I'd note that some companies make extra concentrated fish oils, typically containing about double the EPA/DHA content (and generally costing about twice as much). The main benefit would be less pills to swallow, and a few less calories. For the most part, I think taking 10 standard one-gram fish oil capsules is sufficient. Depending on a dieters meal frequency (discussed below), this should allow 2-3 fish oils capsules (or a teaspoon of liquid fish oil) to be consumed with each meal.

Sort of tangentially, as mentioned in the exercise chapter, athletes may want to take five grams of a fast acting carbohydrate (you can actually buy glucose pills in the diabetic section of any pharmacy) about five to ten minutes before their weight workouts, this will raise blood glucose back to the normal range and help to maintain exercise training intensity. It only adds 20 calories to the daily diet. Again, up to 15-30 grams of carbs (think Gatorade) can be sipped on during a workout, adding 60-120 calories to the diet. While this may slow weight or fat loss slightly, the improvement in ability to maintain training intensity (a key in maintaining LBM) more than makes up for this.

Outside of that one situation, basically all other foods are off-limits on the rapid fat loss diet. No starches, no starchy vegetables, no peanut butter or other fat sources. Nothing. You get to eat protein, vegetables, and your EFAs. The only other things you should consume are fluids and a few select supplements.

A large water intake should be a part of any diet for a variety of reasons. The first is that the body needs fluid on a daily basis (although some of this is obtained from the foods that you eat). You can add lemon to it to improve the taste if you don't like it straight. Some research suggests that a large water intake (especially if the water is cold) may cause the body to expend extra calories although this is somewhat debatable (other research has found no such effect).

At the end of the day, drinking *sufficient* water can't ever hurt a diet and it may help. As well, since low-carbohydrate diets (which the rapid fat loss plan is, of course) can cause the body to drop water, getting sufficient fluids is necessary to prevent dehydration. At the same time, don't go nuts. Too much fluid can be as bad as too little, with excess throwing off mineral balance in the body.

Of course, other non-caloric drinks such as coffee, tea, diet sodas, or sugar free drinks such as Crystal light can be consumed during the day. I'd mention that the occasional dieter will swear up and down that Crystal light (or similar drinks) stall their weight or fat loss.

Finally I want to mention some basic supplements which should be a part of any low-carbohydrate diet. The primary group to worry about are the electrolytes, sodium, potassium, and magnesium. All three are lost on a low-carb diet and supplementing them seems to help people avoid fatigue. Three to five grams of sodium (you should liberally salt your food), up to one gram of potassium and 500 mg of magnesium should be supplemented. One option I'd highly recommend is to purchase one of the "Light Salts" which are typically half sodium and half potassium salt. They generally taste just like normal salt but will provide two of the minerals that you need on the rapid fat loss plan.

I want to mention calcium again, in addition to your one to three servings of dairy protein (from fat free cheese, cottage cheese, or a dairy based protein powder) per day, adding 600 mg of supplemental calcium is a good way to ensure adequate calcium intake and may help with fat loss. Calcium citrate appears to be the best form and a supermarket generic should be more than sufficient.

In addition, a one per day multivitamin won't hurt anyone and provides good nutritional insurance for this or any other diet. While many will disagree, I feel that supermarket generics are at least sufficient. They may not use the best quality ingredients but this can be offset by taking two per day (take them with meals, one in the morning and one in the evening).

Obsessive athletes are probably wondering about all of the other stuff that they might take. Glutamine to support the immune system, branched chain amino acids (which are useful but only at prohibitively expensive doses), leucine, etc., etc. Your call, I don't think most of it is necessary with the levels of protein intakes I'm suggesting but they are all workable and may have a small benefit for the very lean. Frankly, Category 1 dieters who have followed my exact recommendations have yet to report muscle or strength loss, even without using anything exotic supplement wise. I'd also note that protein based supplements such as glutamine, the BCAAs, etc. are all discussed in detail in my recently published The Protein Book as well.

Beyond those few, there are myriad dozens, if not hundreds, of other supplements aimed at fat loss. Some of them have minor effectiveness. Most are over hyped crap. Frankly, with the exception of what I'm going to talk about next chapter (a supplement so important that it deserves its own chapter), none of them are really necessary or worth including as far as I'm concerned.

Other details: Meal frequency and portion size and meal planning

Now that you have a basic idea of what to eat (lean, carbohydrate-free protein sources, lots of fibrous vegetables, an EFA source, water and a few supplements), let's talk about some other issues related to following the rapid fat loss diet: meal frequency, portioning, etc.

First up is meal frequency. Depending on what type of dieting literature you read, you have probably either seen it asserted that you must eat 5-6 times per day to lose weight (bodybuilding, athletic stuff) or that you should only eat 3 times per day (some of the rest of it).

Frankly, given the same caloric intake and adequate protein, it probably doesn't matter very much at the end of the day. Extremely low meal frequencies (two meals per day) are probably marginally worse than higher but by the time you get to three to four meals per day (again, with plenty of slowly digesting protein from food, or perhaps MPI), there's little to no difference.

In any case, I take a bit more free form approach to it all. The basic issue, as far as I'm concerned, is how many calories you'll be eating per day as this determines what a realistic number of meals per day can or should be.

To tell a lighter female who may be eating 1,200 calories per day that she must eat 6 "meals" per day is ludicrous in my opinion, each "meal" will consist of only 200 calories. This is a few bites of food at best and hardly filling; she might be better eating three or four slightly larger meals spaced further apart.

By the same token, a large individual trying to eat 3,000 calories per day would have to eat some monster meals of 1,000 cal per meal if they only ate three times per day. That person would be better of splitting it into five to six smaller meals. None of which is really relevant to the rapid fat loss plan except as words of general introduction.

Within the context of the diet in this book, most people will be eating somewhere between 400 and 800 calories per day or so (some Category 1, or larger Category 2 and 3 dieters with a lot of lean body mass may end up closer to 1200 calories per day). This takes it far out of the realm of a 6 meal per day plan in the first place.

For most, 3 meals tend to be more realistic unless you want each "meal" to be a few bites of food. Maybe 4 if you're at the high end of the calorie intakes. Now, you may remember from a few chapters back that protein contains 4 calories/gram, meaning that 400-800 calories will represent somewhere between 100 and 200 grams of protein. Divided across three meals, that's somewhere between 33 and 77 grams of protein per meal. Divided across four meals, that's 25 to 50 grams of protein at each meal.

To help put this in perspective, the box below shows typical low-carbohydrate, low-fat protein foods (essentially the same list from above) along with the serving size and amount of protein per serving. Additionally, it shows how much of a given protein source would be required to provide roughly 30 grams of protein.

Food	Serving	Protein/serving	#Servings for 32 grams protein
Beef	1 oz	8	4 oz
Chicken	1 oz	8	4 oz
Fish	1 oz	7	3.5 oz
Egg white	1	3.5	7-8 egg whites
Fat free cheese	1 oz	8	4 oz

Obviously, if you need to obtain more protein per meal, you'll need to scale up the number of servings eaten. If you need less, scale them down. I'd note that 3 ounces of any meat is about the amount that will fit in a cupped palm (it's also about the size of a deck of cards). A typical restaurant portion may be double or triple that (8-12 ounces).

As shown above, 33 grams of protein would represent 4-5 ounces of meat; 50 grams would be 6-7 ounces (two cupped palms), 70 grams is 9-10 ounces (three cupped palms). A regular sized can of tuna typically contains 26-30 grams of protein.

Of course, you can mix and match the above foods to hit your protein goals. An egg white omelet could be made out of 6 egg whites (21 grams of protein) with 2 oz of fat free cheese (16 grams of protein) and would provide 37 grams of protein (throw in some vegetables to plump it up and give it more volume). Again, you can scale the amounts depending on how much you need to eat at any given meal. Three to four ounces of lean chicken (24-32 grams of protein) with an ounce of fat free cheese melted on top (8 grams of protein) would provide 32-40 grams of protein. You should get the idea at this point.

If you choose to go the protein powder route (either by itself or mixed into something else such as a serving of cottage cheese), a typical scoop will contain about 24 grams of protein per so (this can vary quite a bit, read the label). You can make an easy dessert by putting a scoop of protein powder (~24 grams of protein) into one serving of cottage cheese (13 grams of protein), add some fiber powder and non-fat sweetener and make a pudding containing 37 grams of protein.

Hopefully that gives you a starting place in terms of portioning your protein, just divide your daily intake up fairly evenly across 3-4 meals, read a couple of labels to figure out amounts and go to town. Essential fatty acid intake is easy: as I've mentioned you want to take either 10 grams of grams of fish oil capsules per day (take 2-3 with each meal depending on your meal frequency), or an equivalent amount of liquid fish oil. Again, flaxseed oil is not a sufficient substitute for fish oils.

Next up are vegetables. I highly recommend you eat some at every meal; they provide important nutrients, will help to keep you full, and keep you regular. As mentioned, vegetables can pretty much be consumed without limits from the list in the box on page

48. Get creative with your vegetable intakes, make salad with each meal, add vegetables to an egg white omelet or make your own stir-fry with lean protein sources and vegetables.

Finally is everything else and I suspect this is where readers will need the most help. Unfortunately, many of the condiments we are used to using either contain a lot of carbohydrates, fat or both. Ketchup, for example, typically contains a lot of sugar. Mayonnaise is basically pure fat. Most salad dressings either have a lot of carbs, a lot of fat or both.

The box below provides some foods (primarily toppings) that can essentially be eaten without limit on the rapid fat loss plan; they all contain too few calories to worry about

---

Free Foods

Condiments: Lemon juice, all spices, vinegar, mustard, soy sauce, some of the new low-carb condiments (see below), salsa or pico de gallo

Beverages: Water, diet free soda, coffee (no cream or sugar), Crystal light or other sugar free drinks, teas (no sugar), broth/bouillon (good for making soup)

With the explosion of low-carbohydrate foods, there has been an increase in the numbers of toppings that can be used on the crash diet. Although I can't seem to find it anymore, I have seen a low-carb teriyaki sauce with a mere 5 calories per tablespoon. Used on chicken breast or lean red meat with some salad, and you can make a tasty meal easily.

I want to note that many of the low-carb salad dressings are basically pure fat. Once again, I suggest you at least check the labels on anything you're considering, fats and carbs tend to hide everywhere.

Finally note that the foods containing zero (or near zero) net carbohydrates are off-limits. The sugar alcohols being used in these foods are converted, to one degree or another, to glucose in the liver and should be counted as carbohydrates.

Eating out

Shockingly, it's actually not that difficult to eat out and stick to the program that I've just laid out. Simply keep in mind that, at any given meal you need a source of lean protein (preferably containing minimal amounts of carbohydrates and fats), lots of fibrous vegetables, and your small EFA source.

Now, you're not going to find EFAs at a restaurant, you'll have to take them with you. But it's usually trivial at most places to get either lean fish or grilled chicken breast (just make sure to get it without sauces or cheese and cooked without any fat) along with some type of salad or steamed vegetables. Of course, you can't have the croutons, cheese or dressing but it's a salad nonetheless. Get them to bring you an oil and vinegar dressing no the side and only use the vinegar.

Even eating at a fast food place is workable on the rapid fat loss plan. Almost all of them offer some type of grilled chicken sandwich and most offer some type of side-salad these days. Toss the bun of course, but grilled chicken plus salad (again, take your EFAs with you) equals a rapid fat loss plan friendly meal in a second.

Summing up

This chapter is arguably the most important in the book since it explains how to actually set up the rapid fat loss plan diet. The first step was to determine how much dietary protein you should be consuming each day. This was based on your diet category (based on your body fat percentage) and activity level.

With that number calculated, the next step is to simply divide your daily protein across the (generally) three to four meals per day that you'll be consuming. So let's say that you calculate that you should be eating 120 grams of protein per day. Divided across three to four meals per day, that yields an intake of 30-40 grams of protein at each meal. Let's say that you're going to eat 40 grams of protein at each of three meals per day.

Either using food labels, or the chart I've provided above, you would then determine what combination of protein foods will meet those goals. For example, you might choose to consume 4 oz of lean chicken (32 grams of protein) with 1 oz of fat free cheese melted on top (8 grams of protein) to get 40 grams. I provided other examples above.

To that protein, the only required nutrient you need is an EFA source. As discussed above, 10 standard one-gram fish oil capsules, or an equivalent amount of liquid fish oil is what I recommend. Ideally, you should take your EFAs with each meal, 2-3 capsules or roughly a teaspoon of liquid fish oil.

While not required, I highly recommend you consume some type of fibrous vegetable with every meal. This can be eaten as salad or worked into your lean protein somehow (e.g. vegetables added to an omelet, make stir fry). Vegetables can also be eaten for snacks between meals.

You should ensure that you get plenty of fluids, this means straight water or any of the non-caloric drinks I listed in the box above. A basic multivitamin along with extra calcium, sodium, potassium and magnesium is also a very good idea. You can use light salt (which is ½ sodium and ½ potassium) on your foods as well.

Metabolic slowdown and what to do about it

The next issue I want to talk about is that of metabolic slowdown on a diet. Once again, this is one of those hideously complicated topics that one day, I should write an entire book about. Here, you're getting the very abbreviated version. This chapter will also act as a bridge for me to talk about what may be the single most important supplement on the crash diet as well as acting as a bridge for the next chapters.

Body weight regulation

Decades of research have led to one rather depressing conclusion: human body weight is regulated. Now what does that mean? To explain it I'm going to use the rough analogy of a thermostat which acts to regulate the temperature of your house. So you set the thermostat at 70 degrees. Now, the thermostat has a meter in it that tells it what the actual temperature of the house is; if the temperature falls below 70, the heat comes on, if temperature goes above 70, the air conditioning comes on.

The human body acts similarly but, in this case, the regulator is the hypothalamus (a structure in your brain) and things such as metabolic rate, hunger, activity levels and hormones are what change when you gain and lose weight. So the hypothalamus is keeping track of your body weight (more accurately, how much body fat you are carrying) and also manages to track how much you're eating (I'll explain how in a second). For the most part, your body wants to keep you where you are at body weight/body fat wise.

So when you start dieting, eating less and losing body weight, your hypothalamus senses it and your body slows metabolism, increases your hunger/appetite levels, and alters hormone levels in a generally negative fashion. To a much lesser degree, when you overeat and start gaining weight, your hypothalamus increases metabolic rate, decreases your hunger/appetite, and ramps up certain hormones.

As I discuss in much more detail in my booklet Bromocriptine the system is very asymmetrical and the human body generally defends against weight loss far better than it does against weight gain. Basically, it's much easier for most people to gain weight than to lose it. There are a small percentage of people who have trouble gaining weight but they are in the minority.

How the body does this: The very, very short course

Explaining the systems involved in body weight regulation would truly take a book and all I really want to say is that there are a number of hormones including leptin, insulin, ghrelin, peptide YY (some of which you may have heard of and others you'll think I'm making up) and others that "tell" your hypothalamus both how much you're eating and how much body fat you're carrying.

All of these hormones respond both to food intake and how much weight/fat you have on you and act as the signals which tell the brain what's going on so that it can make adjustments. A much more detailed description of this system is found in either my Bromocriptine booklet or in The Ultimate Diet 2.0. But, unless you're just interested, you really don't need to know the details.

So when you start a diet, eating less and losing weight, your body notices it and starts to adjust metabolism downwards. Appetite/hunger tend to go up and many hormones change. In essence, this is the "starvation response" that everybody tends to talk about. Metabolism (and weight/fat loss) slow and you get so hungry that you tend to break your diet, frequently eating so much that you put the weight you lost right back on.

I should mention right here that the degree to which this occurs depends a lot on the body fat level of the person in question. Someone at 10% body fat will tend to have far greater issues with this than someone who is at 40% body fat. Keep this in mind as it helps to explain the differences in frequency of free meals, refeeds and full diet breaks discussed in the next chapters.

Metabolic rate reduction: The body weight component

First let me mention that there are two distinct components to the drop in metabolic rate. The first is simply a function of losing body weight. I haven't talked much about metabolic rate, but the amount of calories you burn both at rest and during daily activity tends to be related directly to your body weight: a heavier individual burns more calories than a lighter individual both at rest and during activity (if you don't believe me, try walking a mile with a 20 pound backpack on and see how much harder it is). So as you lose weight, your energy requirements go down.

On which note, I've wondered for a while if it wouldn't be a good dieting strategy to use a weighted vest or backpack to maintain your "effective" body weight, that is replace the lost body weight with weight on the vest/backpack to try to maintain daily caloric expenditure. The effect wouldn't be monstrous, mind you, as wearing the pack would

56

only affect calorie burn during activity (not rest) but every little bit can help at the end of a diet. It's also nice feeling bulletproof because of the weighted vest you're wearing. You will get funny looks from people.

Obviously, short of my backpack/vest idea, there's not much you can do about this component (other than get fat again); if you've reduced your body weight, you will have reduced the number of calories your burn each day because of it. This is another potential role for exercise, especially at the end of the diet, helping to compensate for the reduction in calorie expenditure that occurs as a consequence of losing weight.

Metabolic rate reduction: The adaptive component

But in addition to the reduction in caloric expenditure due solely to weight loss, there is another component called the "adaptive component'. Its existence has been debated over the years with some studies saying it exists and others not. So what is an adaptive component anyway? In this context it means that the body has reduced (in the case of dieting) or increased (in the case of overeating) caloric expenditure more than you'd expect based on the change in body weight.

That is, say that a reduction in weight of 10 pounds would be predicted to lower daily calorie expenditure by 150 calories, but when you measure it, the reduction is actually 250 calories. That extra 100 calories/day reduction is the adaptive component. I want to mention that the adaptive metabolic rate is never sufficient to completely eliminate weight loss; it simply reduces the effective daily deficit (which may slow weight loss).

Perhaps the largest reduction in metabolic rate recorded is of the order of 30-40% (and that was seen in relatively lean men who underwent semi-starvation for months) and most of that drop in metabolic rate was due to weight loss with perhaps 15% of it coming from the adaptive component. Considering that the daily deficit on the crash diet will be 50% or more of daily energy expenditure, the slowing of metabolic rate will not be able to eliminate weight/fat loss, only slow it somewhat.

I should mention that the adaptive component tends to be quite variable and several factors affect it. One is body fatness, generally the fatter someone is, the less of a problem there tends to be with an adaptive decrease in metabolic rate. Tangentially, this probably explains why some studies don't find an adaptive component; they are looking at extremely obese individuals.

Gender also has an effect, women's bodies tend to fight back harder and faster than men's (see my booklet Bromocriptine for more details on this), dropping metabolic rate more than men. This is one of several reasons men typically lose weight and fat faster than women. There is also good old genetic variability; some people's bodies seem to fight back harder and faster than others. Generally, the people who gain weight the easiest lose it the slowest and vice versa.

And what causes the adaptive component of metabolic rate reduction? Primarily the hormones I mentioned above. Actually, not so much those hormones as the systems that they control such as nervous system output, thyroid hormone, and a couple of others. Although you've probably read that levels of thyroid hormone are the primary regulator of metabolic rate, this is an altogether simplistic explanation (even for this book). Rather, the adaptive component of metabolic rate reduction is an integrated response to decreased nervous system output (which is often below normal in obesity to begin with, a metabolic "defect" if you will), thyroid hormone (which may be low to begin with), leptin, insulin and others. When you diet, it simply turns out that all of those systems decrease below normal, causing the adaptive decrease in metabolic rate.

However, the different systems (the main ones I'm going to focus on here are nervous system output and thyroid) have different effects over different time frames. Thyroid, for example, is a fairly long-acting hormone. For example, even if thyroid drops, it can take several weeks for any effects to be seen. I should note that thyroid also has somewhat minor, short-term effects on metabolic rate).

In the short-term, a few days to a few weeks of dieting, the main system that is decreasing metabolic rate is a decrease in sympathetic nervous system (SNS) output. In fact, within 3-4 days of extreme dieting, SNS output can and will drop, lowering metabolic rate slightly (by perhaps 5%). Interestingly, nervous system output actually increases during the first few days of extreme dieting, probably to help mobilize fatty acids for fuel. As well, SNS output and thyroid levels are synergistic, they make each other work better; a drop in SNS output means that thyroid hormones won't have as great an effect as you'd expect.

Since the rapid fat loss program is mostly short-term only (the only people who might stay on it longer than a few weeks are Category 3 dieters for whom the adaptive component isn't as big of a deal in the first place), the only system we are going to concern ourselves with is SNS output. Since, short of using thyroid drugs (or hoping that one of the thyroid boosting supplements on the market actually works) you can't do much about thyroid anyhow (well, see next chapter), there's nothing to be gained worrying about it.

Ephedrine and caffeine: Killer of millions or the ultimate diet pill?

So what about SNS output? Is there any way to increase it? The answer is yes and the compound is cheap, readily available (although less so than it used to be) and safe as long as you use it correctly. That compound is the much maligned (in the over hyped news media) combination of ephedrine and caffeine (known in most circles as the EC stack).

Now, those of you who are currently freaking out in an "EC kills people and Lyle is the devil for talking about it" way need to step back, take a breath, and untwist your panties. Let's talk some facts and all I ask is that you hear me out (people who know that the media hype over the dangers of EC is just hype can skip this section).

The fact is that the EC stack has been clinically studied and used for nearly 2 decades. It has been shown to increase metabolic rate, blunt hunger, may correct the SNS defect present in obesity-prone individuals, increases fat loss and decreases muscle loss on a diet. At least one study suggests that the effects of EC increase over time, as opposed to most drugs which show a decrease in effect with regular use. Recent studies have shown that the herbal forms (ephedra/MaHuang and various herbal forms of caffeine) are equally well tolerated and effective. That's the good news.

However, EC is a stimulant and that means that it has side effects including increased heart rate, blood pressure, jitteriness, and a couple of others. Guess what, all drugs have side effects. Do note that the side effects of EC typically go away within days to weeks of regular use. So what of all of those negative reports, deaths and the rest? Well, like ANY drug you care to name some people should not use EC. Perhaps more to the point with so many things, many people abuse EC.

Ephedrine was a component of many of the herbal Ecstasy compounds years ago so rave kids were using it along with alcohol and who knows what else, several died. As well, many dieters fall into a "More is better" trap with such products, increasing the dose and getting into problems. They figure that if a standard dose causes some weight loss, double or triple the dose should cause double or triple the weight loss. Which it does, but only because death is a way to lose weight very rapidly.

Some people have preexisting health problems such as high blood pressure or cardiac arrhythmias that preclude the use of EC; when people ignore such warnings (as crazed dieters often do), they get into problems. A very real problem is that obese individuals commonly have high blood pressure to begin with; the group that could benefit the most from using EC often shouldn't be taking it.

Basically, like any other drug you care to name, EC tends to be very safe and effective when used intelligently and in a controlled fashion (as it always is in clinical studies) and can be extremely dangerous if you do dumb things like take three times the recommended dose or stack it with other drugs or the types of things that many people tend to do. Once again, this doesn't differentiate it from any drug you care to name, that the FDA has cracked down on herbal ephedra diet pills probably has more to do with politics than anything real.

If you want more facts or don't believe what I'm saying, I highly suggest you surf over to

http://www.drumlib.com

as he has amassed perhaps the most complete account of the EC stack to be found. And if you're still not convinced or aren't interested in EC, you should just turn to the next chapter.

In any event, the extreme caloric deficit of the crash diet makes SNS slowdown a very real issue. Although, as stated above, the adaptive metabolic rate drop can never completely eliminate the deficit (especially when it is this large), using a compound like EC still helps to keep things humming along. The appetite blocking and muscle sparing/fat loss increasing effects are an added bonus. Note that the drop in insulin/SNS output and loss of water on the rapid fat loss diet tends to reduce blood pressure to begin with (which is a good thing if you have high blood pressure and can make you lightheaded if you don't, or run a low blood pressure to begin with), meaning that EC should be *reasonably* safe for most rapid fat loss dieters.

Still, before considering using the EC stack, you need to ask yourself very seriously if you have any preexisting problems (such as cardiac abnormalities, high blood pressure or heart rate or simply a general intolerance to stimulants) that would prevent you from using the EC stack. I don't need someone dropping dead because they chose to take a compound they simply shouldn't have been using in the first place.

Even assuming the answer is no, you're not aware of any reason not to use the EC stack, if you've never used the stack before, I strongly (STRONGLY) suggest that you start with a low-dose and assess your tolerance. But let me back up a bit.

Dosing the EC stack

The rather standard dose of EC for dieting purposes is 20 mg ephedrine (or the herbal equivalent) and 200 mg of caffeine (or the herbal equivalent) taken three times per day. This is what has been used in the clinical research and shown to have the greatest effect on caloric expenditure. Note that some studies suggested the addition of aspirin (making it an ECA stack) would improve the effect. But this was only shown for obese individuals and taking 300 mg of aspirin three times per day is a good way to burn a hole in your stomach/get an ulcer. Whether lower doses of aspirin (say the 81 mg children's size) would have the same effect is unknown.

But, again, if you've never used the EC stack before, jumping straight to the above dose (20/200 three times per day) is a recipe for disaster. DO NOT DO IT unless you have used EC before and know you can tolerate it. Rather, start with a half dose, 10 mg of ephedrine and 100 mg of caffeine taken once per day and see how you react. If you have no problem, move to a full dose taken once per day. If you have no problems there, you can add a second dose, then a final third dose.

In general, you should make sure your last dose of ephedrine comes no later than about 6 hours before your normal sleeping time (i.e. no later than 4pm if you normally go to sleep at 10pm); the stimulant effects keep many people up. So you might take a dose at 8am upon awakening, at 12 pm, and again at 4pm (assuming a 10pm sleep time). Just spread the three doses throughout the day, assuming you can tolerate all three. Note again that the stimulant effects tend to decrease with regular use (so do the appetite blunting effects, unfortunately) but the calorie burning effects continue unabated with at least one study suggesting that they increase with regular use.

Other thermogenics: Norephedrine, synephrine and yohimbe

In the wake of the ephedra ban (note: only the herbal ephedra was banned, ephedrine HCL can still be found at most pharmacies in compounds such as Bronkaid), many companies have tried to bring non-ephedra thermogenics (thermogenesis just means burning calories for heat which is much of what the EC stack does) to market. Almost without exception, they are crap, full of half-effective (or ineffective) compounds that do almost nothing. Even prior to that various companies tried to bring other thermogenics to the market such as norephedrine (the main ingredient in Dexatrim). While an excellent appetite suppressant, norephedrine is not thermogenic in humans as two studies have clearly shown. It is, however, thermogenic in rats so if you have a pet rat with a weight problem...

A substance with some potential utility is synephrine which may improve metabolism and nervous system output (although through a totally different mechanism than ephedrine). A dose of 4-20 mg/day spread throughout the day is what's recommended. I should mention that some of non-ephedrine thermogenics contain bitter orange (aka citrus aurantium) which is simply an herbal form of synephrine. It's about the only ingredient in most non-ephedra based thermogenics that might be worth anything.

And then there's yohimbe (or yohimbine HCL which is the drug form), a compound that helps with fat mobilization, especially from stubborn fat areas. The mechanism of action of yohimbe is slightly up to debate. Some research suggests that its effects are mediated through inhibition of one of the hormone receptors on fat cells (the details of this system are in my Ketogenic Diet book and The Ultimate Diet 2.0 book); other data suggest that it works by increasing hormone release from the nerve terminals. In either event, yohimbe seems to particularly help with stubborn fat deposits especially women's hip and thigh fat. Men's abdominal and low-back fat may also benefit. An upcoming project of mine will deal in detail with getting rid of these stubborn fat depots.

But, before you run out and stock up on yohimbe, a couple of things. First is that if you're not already reasonably lean (I'd say Category 1 and *possibly* Category 2) to begin with, yohimbe won't be of much use to you. The body will take fat from the most readily accessible areas first and stubborn fat is stubborn for a reason.

Additionally, yohimbe, especially the herbal form, can cause all kinds of weird side effects. People often report a combination of sweats and chills along with a feeling that their heart is going to come out of their chest when they exercise (yohimbe also improves blood flow to the genitals which can lead to some potential embarrassment at the gym; it does not, contrary to popular belief, affect testosterone levels). Finally, yohimbe is best used prior to aerobic activity (the aerobics are necessary to burn off the now mobilized fatty acids) although it still might have an effect for a lean dieter doing the crash diet without aerobics.

As one major caveat, you should **never** mix EC and yohimbe; in fact, you shouldn't take them within about 4 hours of one another. The reason is that the side effects of each will multiply and both blood pressure and heart rate can really jump.

If you decide to use yohimbe (again, the yohimbine HCL form is the better choice; less side effects) the effective dose would be 0.2 mg yohimbe per kilogram of body weight or about 0.1 mg per pound consumed with 100-200 mg of caffeine. This would be taken 30-60 minutes before low-intensity aerobic activity (preferably first thing in the morning before eating). So a 150 lb dieter would get just under 15 mg of yohimbe. As with EC it's a good idea to start with a half-dose to assess your tolerance. If you are also using the EC stack, your doses should be taken no closer than 4 hours to the dose of yohimbe/caffeine. So you could do a yohimbe/caffeine combo at 7am prior to morning aerobics and take EC at noon and 4 pm.

61

62

Free meals, refeeds and diet breaks

Ok, so now you're ready to go, you've got your diet set up, know what you're supposed to eat, how much to exercise, and what supplements/other stuff you should be taking. There are a few final issues to deal with; this chapter is the bridge to them.

I want you to try to remember way back in the foreword where I warned you that I'd give some rather specific recommendations on how long you can (or should) stay on a crash diet. That's part of what this chapter is about and I really want you take my recommendations in this chapter to heart: trust me when I say that you ignore them at your own risk.

The other part of this chapter deals with an aspect of dieting that I suspect few of my readers are familiar with, the idea of taking planned breaks from a diet. I'm going to discuss three different approaches, the free meal, the structured refeed and the full diet break. The concept of the full diet break will lead into into a 5-chapter discussion of how to end the crash diet and move to maintenance.

How long to stay on the diet

This ties in with the information on metabolic slowdown that I presented in the last chapter. As I made reference to, how hard and how fast metabolism tends to crash on a diet depends on a lot of factors including gender and genetics (neither of which we can control). But one of the main ones is initial body fatness: fatter individuals can usually diet longer without needing a break from the diet (both a psychological and physiological break) than leaner individuals. So once again your diet category will determine how long you can and/or should stay on the crash diet: the lower the category, the less time you should be on the diet before taking a break of some sort.

What do you mean by a break?

Many readers may be confused as to what I mean by taking a break from a diet. That's because most diet books seem to believe the dieters just sort of stay in this extended diet period forever. If they give guidelines for maintenance, they are usually somewhat vague; you're often just supposed to eat more of whatever the diet in question includes.

Additionally, many dieters, both within the bodybuilding community and in the general public, fall into the trap of confusing dieting harder with dieting smarter. The idea that a planned diversion from the diet (which can last from a single meal to 2 weeks depending on the circumstances) can actually make the diet **work better** goes against their intuition and common sense. With a few exceptions, it's absolutely true. This topic is discussed in more detail in the book that I released at the same time as this one, A Guide to Flexible Dieting. You're going to get sort of an abridged version below but anybody interested more in the topic should pick up that book.

Studies repeatedly show that flexible dieters, that is individuals who allow some flexibility in their eating habits, tend to do better with their dieting efforts, weigh less and succeed more often than rigid dieters (dieters who think that they must adhere to the diet 100% or it's failed). Please read that again: the stricter you are with your diet (i.e. the more absolutist you are), the more likely it is to backfire on you. I imagine most of you have been there, you're cranking away on your diet, you have that one cookie or slip-up, figure that your diet is ruined and consume the whole bag out of guilt. Anything worth doing is overdoing and that's how most people deal with diet slip-ups.

But ultimately this is a self-defeating attitude. A single cookie (or even a single meal) can't undo a week or more of dieting. To use the standard hackneyed cliché: even the greatest baseball players only get a hit 50% of the time if they are lucky (or good). Similarly, Psychologists often refer to a concept called the 80/20 principle which says that as long as you get a given behavior right 80% of the time, the other 20% isn't so important.

Yet dieters often see anything less than 100% perfection as utter failure. Well, rigid dieters do anyhow. Which is probably a big reason why flexible dieters, those folks who are more relaxed about their diet, tend to do better in the long run. Of course, you can't be too relaxed, that's what made you fat in the first place. It's simply a matter of balance: taking that occasional slip-up in stride and not worrying about it too much.

More interestingly, in one recent study, dieters were forced to take 2 weeks off their diet and eat "normally'. The study was trying to find out why dieters fall off the diet bandwagon and figured that was best done by making the dieters include the time off. But what they found was just the opposite: the dieters didn't gain significant weight back and had no problems going back on the diet when the two weeks were up. The diet didn't fail because of the two weeks off although the study did (failed to do what it set out to do).

The researchers weren't absolutely sure why this occurred but it seems likely that by planning the 2 weeks off (rather than letting it be "accidental" as is often the case during a diet), the dieters interpreted the break differently from a psychological perspective. That is, rather than see the 2 weeks as a failure of their own willpower, they saw it as part of the overall plan. This took a potential negative and made it into a positive by changing how the dieters interpreted the break period. This is important and I entreat you to read the previous couple of paragraphs again as they may go the most against your ingrained beliefs about dieting.

Several years ago, I took this concept farther; basically mandating regular refeeds on a diet. To be honest, this wasn't anything new, previous diets had used a similar concept; I just formalized it and hammered out some of the details. Not only did this provide a psychological break on the diet, it helped physiologically by helping to upregulate some of the systems that crash when you diet (discussed in the last chapter and in my previous 2 books).

As well, since the refeeds were part of the overall diet plan, the normal negative "Oh, I blew my diet again, I might as well eat that box of cookies." response was avoided. People started thinking in terms of "Deliberate refeeds to upregulate metabolic rate" (or however they ended up expressing it). Making the break part of the plan took it from being a negative to a positive outcome: it also put dieters in control of the breaks (although, as I'll mention below, some dieters try to abuse what the break is supposed to be).

So with that background out of the way, I'm going to describe three different categories of breaks ranging from the simplest/shortest to the most complicated/longest, each of which will be used in one way or another depending on which diet category you're in. Those three categories are free meals, structured refeeds, and full diet breaks.

Free meals

Just as it sounds, this is a single meal that breaks your diet. When I say break I mean that it doesn't conform to the rest of the diet in either the amount or types of foods you get to eat. The main benefit is psychological, dieting nonstop for days or weeks on end gets to be a real mental grind, more so on an extreme diet like this one.

Knowing that there is light at the end of the tunnel, that a couple of times per week you can eat more or less "freely" goes a long way in helping to keep your sanity. You know that you're never more than a few days away from a free meal which makes those days of dieting far more tolerable. Also, if you have any sort of a social life (family or what have you), a free meal gives you the ability to eat with everybody else and not be a huge pain in the ass because of your current diet.

Now, before you stop reading and go out and start gorging, let's talk about what a free meal is and is not. A free meal is NOT a deliberate attempt to see how much food you can stuff down your gullet although this is how it is commonly interpreted. Invariably people fall out of one psychological trap (that breaking the diet in the first place is a negative) and into another (they try to see how much junk they can gorge themselves on during their breaks). Both cause problems. So don't decide that you're going to try and put down the entire pizza (or two), or bankrupt the all you can eat buffet on your free meal; that's a complete and utter abuse of what the free meal is supposed to accomplish.

Rather, go eat a "normal" meal where you are not supremely obsessed with the content. Don't get me wrong, striving to make healthier choices at this point is always a good thing (especially if you have long-term weight loss maintenance as a goal) but breaking your diet a little bit isn't going to kill you. Want to have some French fries, or a dessert, or just some of the bread or starches that you can't eat on this diet, go ahead. Just don't order two entrees, three desserts eat the entire loaf of bread with butter and half of your spouses dinner and then hit the ice cream place on the way home, call that a "meal" and think I somehow gave you permission to do so.

I think, under most circumstances, a free meal is best eaten out of the house, at a restaurant. You're less likely to go nuts with your total food intake at a restaurant (unless you go to an all you can eat buffet which I strongly discourage). You won't order three desserts (unless you want funny looks from the wait staff and your friends) or eat three meals, which is a real possibility if you eat this meal at home. Also, the going out aspect of the meal gives it more of a reward type of flavor, a special treat for your dieting efforts.

I also think it's best to make the free meal a dinner meal. This is mainly about getting back into the swing of the diet. If you make your free meal lunch or breakfast, it can be psychologically difficult to go back to an extreme diet for the rest of the day. If you make it dinner, by the time you wake up in the morning, you should be ready to get back into your normal dieting rhythm. If you're on an exercise program, especially weight training, it would be ideal to put the free meal on a day when you exercised, this helps ensure that the calories and nutrients in that meal go preferentially towards your muscle instead of into body fat.

As above, it would probably be ideal if you at least kept up some of the parameters of the diet, mainly ensuring some type of lean protein and some veggies. So start with a salad (this helps fill you up a bit so you'll be less likely to pig out) and pick some type of protein (lean is preferred, but a fattier steak is ok too) with your main meal. The main difference is that you can have extra stuff as well with the meal. A baked potato, or bread rolls, or pasta on the side, or fries (not one of each), stuff like that. Dessert (only one serving) is ok too.

Some previous approaches to the free meal concept (for example The Carbohydrate Addicts Diet by the Hellers) have further limited the free meal to one hour in duration. Such a limit may be helpful if it keeps you from turning what should be one meal into a several hour graze (and then rationalizing that it was only one "meal'). At the same time, don't fall into the trap of seeing how much food you can eat in an hour if you do this. I've known of folks who literally start a stopwatch and see how much they can eat in an exact one-hour span (they take it further during structured refeeds, described below). Then they wonder why they aren't losing fat.

I want to give you one warning: do not be surprised if your body weight spikes a little bit the next morning, especially if you eat a lot of carbohydrates at your free meal. Just realize that it is water weight and will drop off shortly after returning to the crash diet. Obviously if you were using the rapid fat loss program to get into shape for some specific event, you wouldn't want the free meal the night before (i.e. save the free meal for the wedding reception or drinks at your high school reunion and enjoy the comments about how good you look while you're eating and drinking freely).

I'll go ahead and mention now that both Categories 2 and 3 get free meals at some point during the week but Category 1 dieters do not. The reason is that Category 1 dieters will only be on this diet for a very short period of time (see below), making free meals both unnecessary and nonproductive. Category 1 dieters also finish their stretch on the crash diet with the longest structured refeed (2-3 days), making a free meal that much less useful. I suppose if Category 1 dieters really needed it (psychologically), they could do one free meal about halfway through their diet. Since, as you'll see below, they are only following the rapid fat loss plan for 10-11 days in the first place, it really shouldn't be necessary.

Structured refeeds

The next "level" up from free meals are structured refeeds, basically deliberate periods of high-carbohydrate overfeeding that are performed from anywhere from 5 hours (at the shortest) to roughly one day (probably the average) up to three days (for example, my Ultimate Diet 2.0). Although a structured refeed has psychological benefits similar to the free meals, it has additional physiological benefits that the free meal lacks.

One of these is the refilling of muscle glycogen (carbohydrate stored within the muscle) which is important for individuals involved in high-intensity exercise performance. Structured refeeds also turn off diet-induced catabolism (roughly: tissue breakdown), helping to spare LBM loss. Done properly, structured refeeds can be used to rebuild muscle lost on a diet. Again, see my Ultimate Diet 2.0 for a lot more details.

Finally, deliberately overeating carbohydrates helps to normalize the hormones I talked about back in the chapter on metabolic slowdown: leptin, ghrelin, insulin, etc. I should mention that it is somewhat debatable whether short refeeds (1 day or less) have much of an impact on metabolic rate although a recent study (in rats, unfortunately) suggests that it does help.

So how does one do a structured refeed? Unfortunately, it depends on a lot of variables that aren't relevant to this book, initial body fat level, how much training you're doing and others all determine how long of a refeed should be done and how often it should be done. In my A Guide to Flexible Dieting, I discuss three different lengths of refeed (from 5 to 24 hours) and all of the details inherent to each. Before I talk about durations and amounts of refeeds in this book, first I want to discuss what foods to eat on the refeed.

Ideally, the refeed will consist primarily of starchy carbohydrates (breads, pasta, bagels, etc) with moderate amounts of protein (simply maintain your normal protein intake) and relatively low amounts of fat. You can consume a small amount of "junk food", high sugar items such as candies or fat free yogurt or ice cream or what have you. Of course, fruit is also a good choice. But most of your carbohydrates should come from starchy foods. You can also increase dietary fat over your normal diet intake during the refeed but keep it limited, a maximum of 50 grams of dietary fat over the 5-hour span. That's not much fat, three to four tablespoons of peanut butter, for example.

Essentially, doing a refeed on the rapid fat loss plan is as simple as eating your normal meals containing protein, EFAs and vegetables and then adding a bunch of starchy carbohydrates to hit the numbers above.

I'd mention that, optimally, a refeed would come around a resistance training workout (this will tend to shuttle the incoming carbohydrates into the muscles) and preferably in the evening with the refeed ending at bedtime. During the day, simply eat your normal dieting meals up until you begin the refeed. So if you normally lift weights at 6pm, you would start by having a moderate sized meal containing carbohydrates, protein and fat about an hour beforehand (at 5pm). Train and then plan on consuming the remainder of your refeed calories/carbs from immediately following the workout until you go to bed. If you train from approximately 6 to 7pm, eat a big carb meal at 7pm, and another at 9pm. You would aim to get your target carbohydrate amounts from 5pm to 10pm. The next morning, it's right back to the rapid fat loss diet plan.

So how long and how often should a refeed be done? As mentioned above, this depends on several variables; main one I'm going to consider here is what dieting category you're in.

Category 3 dieters are the simplest, they don't get refeeds, they only get free meals and full diet breaks (discussed further below) in-between phases of active dieting.

Category 2 dieters will be performing a 5-hour refeed once per week during the diet (they also get one free meal per week). During their refeed, they should try to consume 1.5-3 grams of carbohydrate per pound of LBM (~3-6.5 g/kg for the metrically inclined). So a Category 2 dieter with 150 pounds of LBM would consume between 225 and 450 grams of carbohydrates (900-1800 calories worth) in that 5-hour time span. While this may seem like a lot (and it certainly will be compared to the rapid fat loss diet itself), it's actually not that much compared to the rather high intake of carbohydrates in the modern diet in the first place. A medium sized bagel may have 50 grams of carbohydrates or so; consuming 4 of them would provide 200 grams of carbohydrates.

That's a pretty big range, mind you and how many carbs a Category 2 dieter should eat during the refeed will depend on the amount of exercise (weight training) they are doing. If you're weight training on the rapid fat loss plan, target the high value of 3 grams per pound for the refeed. If you're not weight training (either not exercising at all or only doing aerobic activity), target the 1.5 grams per pound value.

For Category 1 dieters, I recommend ending the rapid fat loss stint with a relatively long refeed of 2-3 days before either moving to maintenance or returning to dieting. My Ultimate Diet 2.0 used a 3 day refeed comprised of 12-16 grams of carbs per kilogram (about 5-6 grams per pound) on the first day, about half of that (2-3 g/lb) on the second day, and about half (1-1.5 g/lb) of that on the third day. This should be more than sufficient for a Category 1 dieter ending the rapid fat loss plan. The third day could probably simply be dropped as well.

As a final comment about refeeds, do be forewarned that body weight can spike significantly after a structured refeed, from glycogen and water storage. A five to ten pound gain in one day is not uncommon (it's the same five to ten pounds you dropped right off the bat rapidly). As with the free meal, the water weight drops back off within a couple of days of returning to the crash diet.

Full diet break

And finally is the full diet break, a period of 1-2 weeks where the dieter goes back to eating at maintenance. With the exception of Dan Duchaine (who recommended that a 10 week contest diet cycle be broken up into 4 weeks of dieting, 2 weeks off, and 4 weeks of dieting) and myself, I don't recall this suggestion being made in popular dieting literature. But, for a variety of reasons (the study mentioned above included), it makes a tremendous amount of sense to include a full break within the context of longer dieting periods.

Let's face it; dieting for long periods at a stretch becomes a real psychological drag. Admittedly the crash diet avoids some of this by being more extreme for a shorter period of time. Even then, for someone who is extremely overweight or over fat, it may take several months before all of the weight desired is lost. Expecting someone to diet strictly for that time period is simply unrealistic. Breaking the diet up into more manageable stretches, 8-12 weeks at a time with a 2 week break makes the whole process much easier psychologically, as no individual dieting period lasts all that long without a break.

Full diet breaks can also be scheduled to coincide with vacations or special events, giving them that much more utility. Since the break is now part of the diet structure, rather than an occurrence that is out of the dieter's control, the psychological effect is different. As I described above: what was a negative, a failure of willpower, becomes a positive, a structured part of the diet that makes it work better in the long-term. My experience, and the study above, shows that folks who go into diet breaks planning to make them a break (e.g. a vacation) have an easier time getting back on the diet bandwagon when the break is over.

An additional issue is the metabolic slowdown that I described in the last chapter. Although structured refeeds help out somewhat, metabolism eventually slows and progress on the diet slows as well. Taking two weeks off the diet to eat "normally" helps to upregulate metabolic rate (including nervous system output and thyroid hormones), making fat loss occur more efficiently when you go back to dieting. Of course, this is predicated on the fact that you don't regain a tremendous amount of fat back during this period, and that's predicated on the fact that your caloric intake still needs to be kept under control.

So what does it mean to do a full diet break? First let's talk about what not to do. As with the free meals and structured refeeds, the goal of the diet break should not be to see how badly you can eat for 2 weeks or how much junk food you can put into your mouth. Obviously, returning to the eating habits that made you fat in the first place is a mistake as well (see the next chapter). So how does one properly do a full diet break?

The first step is that calories should be adjusted to the maintenance level, that is the caloric intake that will maintain your current weight or body fat. I'll tell you how to do this in the next chapter which is all about maintaining your weight loss. Protein intake should be kept at the same levels as on the crash diet (Category 2 and 3 dieters may want to increase their protein intake slightly as higher protein intakes have been found to limit weight regain after a diet ends); vegetable and essential fatty acid intake should remain the same as well.

The main change is the addition of more carbohydrates and fats (to raise calories to current maintenance). Carbohydrates need to be raised to at least 100 grams per day (more if you're exercising), as this is necessary to upregulate thyroid hormone levels. Dietary fat intake should come up as well, to moderate levels (20-25% of total calories is about optimum). Again, I'll give more details on this in the next chapters. If you're involved in an exercise program while dieting, you should maintain it at some level during the break; if you're not exercising, the break is a good time to start.

About the only group that usually can't even consider taking a full diet break are athletes and contest bodybuilders (maybe models) who are under a very specific time frame to reach their goals: the two weeks of dieting time that they lose may not be justified if they don't get into shape in time for the contest, competition or photo shoot. Of course, I'd mainly argue that they should have started dieting earlier so that they could include a two-week diet break but this doesn't really help them now.

So with the exception of those Category 1 dieters who are under a strict time frame, a full diet break will be applicable for all categories of dieters; all that will change is how often they take a break. As with structured refeeds and the comments I made above: the fatter you are to start with, the longer you can diet without a break. Obviously, if you're only using the crash diet for purely short-term results, to lose weight for a special event, and don't care if you regain all of the weight, then just go back to your old bad eating habits when you're done. Once again, while I don't advocate this, I accept that that is what some people will do. I'll discuss this more next chapter.

Putting it all together

Ok, so let's look at the three diet categories in terms of the maximum time they can or should stay on the crash diet as well as how they'll integrate each of the above three types of breaks into their crash diet. Once again, with the exception of Category 1 dieters who are under a time crunch (who should return to dieting after a 2-3 day structured refeed), a full diet break should be followed at the end of the dieting period. Table 1 explains it all.

Table 1: Frequency and duration of free meals, refeeds and full diet breaks

Category	Full diet break	Free meals	Refeeds
1	Every 11-12 days	No	2-3 full days at the end
2	Every 2-6 weeks	1 per week	5 hours once/week
3	Every 6-12 weeks	2 per week	None

So Category 1 dieters have the fun of going straight through without free meals or refeeds for 11-12 straight days. At which point they should perform a 2-3 days high-carb, high-calorie refeed (as discussed above) prior to going back to normal dieting (a second cycle of PSMF is a possibility although I don't really recommend it). As mentioned above The carb-load guidelines in the Ultimate Diet 2.0 work fine and finishing up the week of dieting with the tension/power workout combo in described there would be a very good idea. Please trust me when I say that trying to follow the rapid fat loss plan for longer than this rather short time period will seriously screw you if you're already lean.

Yes, I know it's tempting to just keep dropping fat like crazy but without some major drugs to deal with metabolic slowdown and muscle loss, this will cause more harm than good.

Category 2 dieters have it easiest in a sense. First and foremost, Category 2 dieters will typically remain on the rapid fat loss plan for anywhere from 2-6 weeks depending on how much fat they have or want to lose. Two weeks is, of course, the minimum, but six weeks is the maximum before a two-week diet break should be taken. Then they can either go back to more "normal" dieting (meaning a more moderate caloric deficit) or perform another run on the rapid fat loss plan (if desired). As well, they get both a free meal and a 5-hour refeed every week.

Category 3 dieters, as a consequence of being fatter, usually have an easier time sticking to the rapid fat loss plan for extended periods. Many have reported that their hunger goes away completely and once they are in the swing of dieting, they have no problem staying with it over the long haul. One of my testers literally followed it for weeks and weeks on end, his motivation come from watching the scale drop daily and he had little problem with hunger or appetite (or energy levels) past the first few days. Two free meals per week should prevent any real psychological problems; simply follow the recommendations as given above.

I have one last comment for Category 2 and 3 dieters which has to do with how the free meals (or free meal/refeed for Category 2) should be scheduled during the week. Ideally, they should be spaced fairly far apart; you don't want to put them on consecutive days such as Friday and Saturday for example. I mean, conceivably, you could really abuse the concept and do them on Saturday and Sunday, then the following Monday and Tuesday. That's two per week, right? Well….yes. But it's not accomplishing what it should be accomplishing.

Rather, space them out across the week. If you have plans to go out with family or friends on a Saturday night, plan one of your free meals (or your refeed) for that night. The other might ideally be placed on a Tuesday or Wednesday so that you get several days of rapid fat loss dieting in-between.

72

Ending the Diet - Introduction

I imagine most dieters are familiar with the statistics showing that something like 90-95% of dieters regain all of the weight that they lost on a diet. Now, there are many reasons that people regain lost weight and fat and it's a topic I cover in greater detail in my book A Guide to Flexible Dieting.

In addition to all of the other myriad reasons people regain all of the lost weight, a big factor is that people seem to think that a diet is short-term only, that once they've lost the weight they can just go back to their old eating habits and somehow not get fat again. While it would be nice if it worked out this way, it doesn't. If you go back to the way that you used to eat (that made you fat in the first place), you'll just get fat again. Which means that, to maintain the weight/fat you've lost, you have to maintain at least some portion of your diet and activity habits.

That's the topic I want to address in the next several chapters, how to move from rapid fat loss dieting into a maintenance phase that can be sustained. In this chapter, I want to make some introductory remarks and, in the chapters after that I'm going to give two different options of how to eat at maintenance.

I should mention that the full diet break mentioned last chapter is ultimately nothing but moving to maintenance for a two week span. That is to say, the information in the next several chapters applies to both the full diet break and moving to long-term maintenance; the difference is only one of duration. First, I want to look at the two most general options for what to do when you're done dieting.

Option one: Go back to your old eating habits and get fat again

While I certainly don't recommend this option, I realize that it's what some people who use this diet (or any diet for that matter) are going to do. This is especially true of those individuals who used the rapid fat loss plan as a purely short-term thing, to drop weight fast for a special event (e.g. wedding, high-school reunion). If you really don't care about getting fat again and want to throw away all of the effort you put into dieting, I can't really stop you. So go back to your old eating habits, get fat and be happy. That's all I have to say about this.

Option two: Move to a maintenance diet

Once again, this ties in with the full diet break I mentioned in the last chapter and represents my preferred option (with a couple of exceptions I'll mention below) for ending a diet: move into a maintenance diet. Before I explain what a maintenance diet, I need to point out something very important.

When moving to maintenance, most people's body weight will increase by a few pounds. This is especially true after a low-carbohydrate diet (such as this one), especially when carbohydrates are reintroduced (which I'm going to be suggesting). This small weight gain simply represents water, electrolytes, increased food in the gut, etc. This weight gain is no big deal and I don't want people to freak out about it. Remember that you probably dropped anywhere from 5-10 (or more) pounds of water weight while on this diet, regaining some should be expected and no big deal.

So what is a maintenance diet? By definition, a maintenance diet is one that will maintain your current body weight or body fat level. Now, it would be unrealistic for you to maintain your body weight with zero fluctuations, changes in water balance and the rest will cause some fluctuations (women all know what can happen to their body weight during different parts of the menstrual cycle).

As well, nobody should expect themselves to eat an exactingly identical amount of food every day while doing an exacting amount of exercise. Ok, maybe obsessed bodybuilders but nobody without that particular psychology can be expected to do it in the long-term. Frankly, being that obsessive tends to be a recipe for failure for most people (see A Guide to Flexible Dieting for more information).

Let's be realistic: nobody is perfect every day of his or her life. More importantly, who wants to get to the end of their life, having had no enjoyment or pleasure, but being able to claim that their body weight never wavered even a bit? Let's relax this a little bit and say that a maintenance diet (and exercise program) will maintain your body weight or body fat within a relatively narrow range, maybe three to five pounds in either direction (with the big concern being an increase). Basically, if your body weight (and this doesn't include the weight gain from moving back to maintenance) starts to climb by more than that three to five pounds, you need to clamp down a bit more on the diet (or get your exercise plan back on track) before things get out of hand.

In this vein, I want to note that studies of successful dieters note many common behavior patterns but one that is relevant to this chapter is regular monitoring of their body weight. That is, successful dieters tend to keep track of their weight (or body fat) on a regular basis. This could be daily or weekly but keeping regular track tells them when they are slipping and regaining the lost weight/fat so that they can buckle down again. You might contrast this to folks who steadfastly avoid the scale (or always make it a point to wear loose fitting clothes) to avoid the realization that they are getting fat (again). Then they wonder how they "woke up" fat one day.

If you don't like the scale or body fat measurement, you can simply pick a particular piece of clothing that represents your goal weight/fat level and try it on every so often. If it's getting tight again, you're slipping and it's time to get back on top of your diet and exercise program to get back where you need to be.

Again, it's unrealistic for someone's weight or body fat to be completely unchanging but you're better off getting back on top of your diet and exercise when you've only gained a few pounds than when you've gained a bunch.

Ok, so back to maintenance. As above, a maintenance diet is exactly that, a diet that contains the number of calories (and fulfills other requirements such as protein and essential fatty acids) that will equal your activity level so that your weight/fat level is more or less stable within some range. That's all I'm going to say about this in this chapter, I'll get into more details in the next several chapters.

A couple of exceptions

Within the context of the diet described in this booklet, the main exception to moving back to maintenance dieting are contest bodybuilders or athletes who used the rapid weight loss diet to get caught back up with their preparation. Since they don't get a full diet break (only a 2-3 day structured refeed at the end of the diet), they don't have to worry about maintenance until after their contest.

For those individuals, trying to maintain contest levels of leanness is unrealistic anyhow. They are going to regain some weight and fat and then move into maintenance (or perhaps focus on adding muscle which means an above maintenance calorie diet).

A second exception to the move back to maintenance is long-term dieters who used a few weeks of crash dieting to kick start their weight/fat loss before moving into a more moderate weight/fat loss diet with a less extreme food restriction. Rather than moving straight back to maintenance, this category of dieters would increase calories to a more reasonable level (rather than the extremely low caloric intake of the rapid weight loss diet) and continue their diet. This is discussed in detail in Chapter 15.

Two different ways to eat at maintenance

For everyone else, moving back to maintenance will either be used during a full diet break (see last chapter if you've forgotten already) or when the diet is (finally) over. I want to mention now that I'm going to describe two different approaches to moving to maintenance in the next several chapters.

The first approach is aimed at people who really hate counting calories (i.e. most of them). While I'm leery of programs that don't impose some sort of portion control (and note that many popular programs simply hide caloric control while having you count exchanges, or points, or what have you), the simple fact is that most people are not going to keep meticulous track of their food on a day-to-day basis. So I'm going to give some general eating guidelines that will *tend* to prevent issues with over consuming calories. I'll simply note that if you find your body weight increasing out of the range discussed above, you're going to have to impose some restriction on yourself.

The second approach is for that small minority who is willing to count calories, or at least keep track of their food intake on some level (whether it's portions or what have you). There's more math to determine your daily intake (which is why I suspect most people won't do it) but I think it gives more overall control. I should note that even readers who plan to use the calculation based method in Chapter 14 should still read the next two chapters, as it covers a great deal of information related to food choices and overall meal planning. I'll make a few additional comments on the topic in Chapter 14 as well.

A mixed approach

One approach I've found that is useful is for people who really hate counting calories/portions to spend some time period (say three to seven days or so) doing so. That means reading labels, getting out the measuring spoons and cups and generally being miserable and obsessed. The reason for this is that most people are simply atrocious at estimating their food intake.

Studies routinely show that people can underestimate their food intake by 50% (and overestimate their activity by 50% as well). It's not that these folks are lying; most people simply have no conception of what a serving of a given food is; this is especially true in our supersized world where food portions keep getting bigger and bigger and bigger. When you get them to actually monitor/measure their food intake, they become far more aware of how much (or little, in rare cases) they are actually eating.

Making folks go through the headache of measuring everything for a few days helps them realize not only how much they're eating but what real world portion sizes are. Once they have that established, they can get away with eyeball estimations of their daily intake.

Which is just a longwinded way of saying that some readers may wish to follow the second approach, calculating their requirements and keeping track of everything for some short period of time. This is simply to get an idea of what portions are and about how much food is actually their maintenance level. Once that is established, they can move back to the first approach and sort of eyeball their food intake.

Once again, the ultimate criterion of whether your current food intake (and activity level) constitutes maintenance is what is happening in the real world to your body weight or body fat. Are your pants getting tighter or is the scale going up? No matter what you think you're eating or how much I've suggested as an estimate of your maintenance, you're clearly eating too much for your activity level and need to scale back your food intake, or increase your activity levels, or both to get your body weight under control.

Moving to maintenance: Fast versus slow

Before I describe the two different approaches to setting up a maintenance diet over the next several chapters, I want to mention that there two different ways to move back to maintenance: fast and slow, which are exactly what they sound like.

In a fast approach, calories are basically ramped up to maintenance quickly over a day or two. This can actually be done in concert with a structured refeed, just make the first day(s) of your refeed the return to maintenance. So start with a 1-2 day period of high-carbohydrate/high-calorie overfeeding as per the guidelines last chapter and then scale back calories to maintenance levels for the duration of the break (or long-term maintenance).

The drawbacks to this option are that it's easy to lose control of food intake (what should be a 1-2 day refeed turns into a week of gorging) and the bloating and water retention can be annoying. Some people also report gastric upset and gas when they ramp up carbs after they haven't been eating any for a while. I think the fast option is probably best for Category 1 dieters (those who aren't under a time crunch) who already have good food control and won't have a problem returning to maintenance after a structured refeed. Category 2 and 3 dieters may still be dealing with changing long-term eating habits and the slow option, described next, is probably better overall.

Which brings us to the other approach to returning to maintenance which is the slow approach. Again, this is exactly what it sounds like; calories are gradually raised to maintenance over some time period (generally a week). Of course, how you go about adding foods back will depend on whether you're using the non-counting/eyeball method described in Chapter 13 or the counting method described in Chapter 14. I'll address this topic individually in each chapter.

I'd say the big advantage of the slow approach is that it avoids major weight spikes which can cause negative psychological effects. The disadvantage is that it's less fun and means you have to be meticulous about your food intake the whole time. However, this can help with food control, many individuals are completely unaware of what their actual food intake is (or how much, or little, food actually represents maintenance levels) and having to be very aware of your food intake on a day to day basis (at least initially) can act as a teaching tool and help with changing long-term eating habits.

Maintenance versus the two-week diet break

To wrap up this chapter, I want to make a couple of concluding comments about the possible differences between moving to maintenance for the long-term versus doing the full diet break that I described in chapter 10. The primary difference, of course, is that moving to maintenance is an attempt to keep weight more or less stable in the long-term. Which isn't to say that further dieting might not be attempted at some later date, it's simply not the major goal.

In contrast, the full diet break is used to break up periods of active dieting, meaning active caloric or food restriction to generate weight or fat loss. For the most part, the difference is only one of time: moving to maintenance is long-term; the full diet break is only 2 weeks. The only real comment I want to make in this regards is that it is crucial that daily carbohydrate intake be at least 100 grams per day during a full diet break (i.e. between periods of active dieting). The reason is that this amount of carbohydrates is necessary to increase levels of thyroid hormone, a critical aspect of up regulating metabolic rate.

Frankly, hitting this amount of carbs should be no real problem whether you follow the non-counting approach described in the next two chapters, or the meticulous calorie counting approach described after that. I've built it into the recommendations so that you don't have to really think about it. I'm only bringing it up in case your general tendency is to skimp on dietary carbs for fear that they will "make you fat'. Compared to normal daily carbohydrate intakes in modern diets, 100 grams is a pittance (a mere 400 calories) and within the context of the other recommendations is nothing to worry about.

Moving to Maintenance: Non-counting Method Part 1

As I mentioned last chapter, I suspect that a majority of readers really don't want to have to count calories on a day to day basis. Certainly not every day for the rest of their life in any event. Towards that end, I'm going to offer an approach to body weight maintenance that doesn't require (much) in the way of calculating or calorie tracking.

In this chapter, I'm going to make some general comments about food intake, appetite and caloric intake and in the next chapter I'll give the actual guidelines for setting up a non-counting based maintenance diet.

Yet another warning

I want to make it very clear upfront that I am leery as hell of approaches that rely entirely on the individual to gauge their food intake without some sort of monitoring. The reason for this is the number of studies that repeatedly show just how bad people are at it. As mentioned last chapter, people can readily underestimate their food intake by up to 50%, while overestimating their activity by the same 50%.

It's no wonder that people are gaining weight while thinking (and swearing up and down) that they eat very little and burn a ton of calories through exercise. Once again, I'm not saying that folks are lying; people are just really bad at estimating things.

Now, a typical solution to this problem (and the one I'm going to take) is to give a set of eating rules that makes it relatively more difficult to overeat. There are a lot of ways to do it and I'm simply going to present one of them. But note my choice of words two sentences back "relatively more difficult". That's not the same as saying that it's impossible to overeat.

As I mentioned previously, human body weight is notoriously well regulated and people can easily find themselves gaining back weight even if they appear to be doing everything correctly. As many dieters who have followed the "You don't have to count calories as long as you eat a certain way" types of diets have found out the hard way, either weight loss stalls, or weight gain restarts.

This is one of the big reasons to regularly monitor at least your body weight or body fat (or measure your waist or use some particular piece of clothing to gauge the fit) semi-regularly: it will alert you to when things are sliding. That is, even if you think that you're not overeating, if the scale is creeping back up or that pair of pants is fitting more tightly, clearly you are in a calorie surplus. That's true even if you follow the guidelines I'm going to give.

This is yet another reason I suggest you spend at least *some time* measuring and weighing foods when you eat them, to get a better idea of what portions actually are relative to what you think they are. I'll mention this below and, unfortunately, make one very serious recommendation about something you really should measure.

How different macronutrients affect spontaneous food intake

Ok, first I should probably define what is meant in the section heading by "spontaneous food intake'. Basically, that phrase refers to the amount of food that people will eat if left to their own devices. That is how much they will eat when they aren't monitoring their food intake at all.

This is an important concept, as different types of foods affect spontaneous food intake differently. With the exception of some of the goofier diet schemes out there, most of the "Eat all you want but don't worry about counting calories" approaches recommend that dieters eat in such a way that spontaneous food intake is automatically reduced.

Quite in fact, this is the basic theory behind both low-fat AND low-carbohydrate diets (I'm ignoring the idea of a metabolic advantage inherent to low-carb diets, that's a can of worms I don't want to address here). Which probably confused the heck out of everyone, so let me explain.

A great many studies have shown that high fat diets (lets ignore the meaninglessness of that term) tend to promote what researchers call passive over consumption of calories. Translated into non-gibberish, that means that when you give people access to high fat foods, they tend to eat more at a given meal without noticing it. Hence passive over consumption. The essential problem is that, in the short-term (i.e. during a meal), fat doesn't blunt hunger or alter food intake.

So the logic goes, if people reduce fat intake, they'll end up eating fewer calories and lose weight. That's it, the whole premise was more or less based around the idea that if people eat less fat, they'll eat fewer calories and lose weight. This wasn't the only reason, mind you, but it was one of the main ones.

And this is true to a small degree although the effect amounts to very little in the long run. It's been estimated that for every 1% reduction in fat intake, you will lose a whopping 1.6 grams of weight per day. Which, over the range that people can realistically reduce fat intake adds up to almost nothing, maybe 5-10 pounds lost over 6 months which is nothing to write home about. This also assumes that people don't just eat more of the other foods. Which turns out to be a rather incorrect assumption in the real world.

Additionally, there's a limit to how far dietary fat can be reduced before the diet tastes like cardboard and people won't follow it (some research has found better dietary compliance for moderate compared to very low fat-diets). As well, people on low-fat diets, just like everyone else, often start to regain weight even if they keep fat intake low. Why? Because they start to eat more of the foods that *are* allowed.

None of this was helped by the fact that when the low-fat craze came about, food companies rushed high calorie but low or nonfat foods (Snackwell's anybody?) to market. Since people figured that all they had to pay attention to was fat intake, they ended up overeating anyway by eating high calorie but low- or nonfat foods.

So how can the same basic idea apply to low-carbohydrate diets? First let me say that numerous studies have shown that spontaneous caloric intake on low-carbohydrate (also called ketogenic diets) goes down. There are a few reasons for this.

Perhaps the primary one is that when you remove an entire category of food (carbohydrates) that happens to make up 50% or more of people's food intakes, they pretty much can't help but eat less.

As well, since protein turns out to have the largest effect on hunger blunting, the high protein intake tended to help as well (as least one researcher thinks that the benefits of low-carb diets are occurring because people typically increase their protein intake on such diets). The fat intake also tends to keep people full in the long run which seems to contradict what I wrote above about spontaneous food intake but I'll explain in a second.

Additionally, for people who don't handle carbohydrates well (because they are insulin resistant), high carbohydrate intakes tend to spike and crash blood glucose, making them feel lethargic and hungry. Low-carbohydrate/higher-protein diets have been shown to stabilize blood glucose in these folks and the blood sugar crash induced hunger goes away. Finally, ketones (which are produced by the liver when carbohydrates are taken below a certain level) may blunt hunger.

Of course, while this works in the short-term, anybody who's been on a low-carbohydrate diet for any period of time realizes that the same type of effect as with low fat eventually occurs. Either weight loss stalls or body weight starts climbing again. This is especially true for people who have bought into the idea that "calories don't count" as long as you are in ketosis. Which would be lovely if it were true, but it's not.

The reasons are similar to what happens on low-fat diets: people start eating more of the foods that they are allowed. As well, the high fat intake of most low-carbohydrate diets can come back to bite people in the ass, unless their appetite really gets blunted, it's altogether too easy to eat a ton of calories (when the foods are very high in fat) and lose no weight or fat.

Finally, companies are now rushing low-carb (but high-calorie) foods to market which is going to lead people down the same road as what happened with low fat diets. Focused only on carbohydrate content, they'll end up overeating and either not lose weight or end up gaining it.

And that's how both low-fat and low-carb diets are predicated on the basic idea that, by altering your food intake, people will spontaneously eat less and lose weight.

Of great interest recently is the impact of dietary protein on spontaneous food consumption. Recent work has shown that increasing dietary protein intake (in one study, subjects increased protein intake from 12% to 25%) causes a spontaneous reduction in caloric intake causing weight and fat loss. Although "high-protein" diets are often pooh-poohed by mainstream nutrition types, the research is clear that consuming more lean dietary protein helps with weight and fat loss. This is one important reason to keep dietary protein high even when moving to maintenance, it tends to help people to keep their food intake under control. Studies also show that less weight is gained (and the weight that is gained tends to be LBM) when protein is kept high during maintenance. I'll discuss this in more detail in a later chapter.

I suppose I should mention alcohol since it is a nutrient (of sorts) that people consume. Unfortunately, the effects of alcohol on spontaneous food intake and body weight are a little bit schizophrenic. In men increasing alcohol intake tends to cause an increase in body weight (measured by BMI); in women, increasing alcohol tends to be associated with a decreased body weight. The physiological reasons for this are still up to debate. A big part of it is that men tend to eat (and eat fatty foods) when they drink while women tend to drink instead of eating.

How nutrients affect satiety and satiation

Ok, I know I threw a couple more big words at you up there so let me explain them briefly. Satiation is basically short-term hunger, over the course of a meal or so; satiety has to do with longer-term hunger (more accurately called appetite). This is an important distinction to make because each of the macronutrients can affects each somewhat differently.

As I mentioned above, dietary fat tends to have almost no effect in the short-term, which is why we get the effect of passive over consumption. In contrast, both protein and carbohydrate tend to blunt hunger in the short-term. Now I want to comment that I think the studies in question are a little bit goofy. Typically, they use what is called a pre-load design, subjects are given a snack (containing various amounts of the nutrients) and then allowed an all you can eat buffet about 30 minutes later. Researchers look at the food intake at the buffet and draw some (in my mind, poor) conclusions about real world food intake.

Ignoring every other issue with these studies, one of the most important is that they only look at a single meal. I bring this up because how much you eat over a span of 24 hours (or days) is far more important than what you eat at a single meal. And how much you eat over a day depends to some degree on how long you go between meals. Ultimately, a study looking at a single meal (especially using a preload design) tells us little about real world eating behavior.

I bring this up because, as anybody who has followed an extremely low-fat diet knows, dietary fat tends to keep you from getting hungry as soon. Readers may be familiar with the idea of a meal that "sticks to their ribs', an old folk saying referring to how long certain foods sit in the stomach. Higher fat intakes (up to a point) make food sit in the gut longer, and that tends to keep people fuller in the long-term.

Within the context of the typical low-fat diet, this is made even more pronounced when the diet is low in fiber (which slows the rate at which food leaves the stomach) and high in refined carbohydrates (the ones that people like to eat). If you combine that with a low-protein intake, the problems are even more compounded. In that situation, you get a lot of carbs hitting the bloodstream very rapidly, first spiking and then crashing blood glucose which tends to promote hunger.

In many dieters, extremely low-fat intakes, especially when they are coupled with a low-fiber, low-protein and highly refined carbohydrate intakes make people hungrier. I want to point out that this has as much to do with an incorrect diet setup as with the concept of the high-carbohydrate diet itself. People who get sufficient protein, and some dietary fat, along with choosing less refined carbohydrates usually do just fine with such a diet. But I digress.

You can easily test this yourself. First eat something like a bagel or some other refined carbohydrate by itself. See how soon you are hungry again. If you're like most people, it will be fairly soon. Now eat that same bagel with ½ to 1 tablespoon of peanut butter on it and see how much longer you stay full. Between the protein content of the peanut butter and the fat content, the entire combination will stay in your stomach longer, promoting fullness. As well, the fat and protein will tend to slow the entry of glucose into the bloodstream, avoiding major blood glucose swings and crashes.

Basically, dietary fat is sort of a double-edged sword when it comes to caloric intake, satiety and satiation. High dietary fat intakes tend to promote excessive caloric intakes via the passive over consumption effect; very low fat intakes tend to leave people hungrier sooner (especially when combined with a diet of highly refined carbohydrates and too little protein and fiber) and they end up eating more as well.

This argues for a moderate fat intake (20-25% of total calories, I'll explain more next chapter) as probably being optimal and some recent research supports that idea; moderate fat diets tend to have better dietary adherence and improve health to a greater degree than extremely low or high fat diets. Moderate dietary fat intakes also appear to give an optimal effect in terms of slowing glucose release into the bloodstream and moderating blood glucose levels.

I already mentioned above that protein has been found to have the greatest impact on hunger. In the short-term studies, carbs come in second and fat is last. Over the longer term, whether carbs or fat is superior sort of depends.

Unrefined naturally occurring carbohydrates *tend* to keep people fairly full, especially when combined with protein, fat and fiber but the more highly refined carbohydrates (i.e. the ones people are actually eating in the real world) often stimulate hunger more often than not. Between a fast rate of digestion and everything that accompanies them, highly refined carbs can cause more problems than they solve.

Moving to Maintenance: Non-counting Method Part 2

In the last chapter, I introduced some general concepts about how protein, carbs and fat can spontaneously affect caloric intake. That directly leads into this chapter which will list some general guidelines and explain how to put it all together to develop a maintenance level diet that doesn't require you to count and measure every morsel of food.

Eating guidelines

After the last chapter, you should already have a pretty decent idea of what I'm going to suggest in this chapter. Below, I'm going to list a series of "rules" for eating that will tend to make strict calorie counting "mostly" unnecessary. It encompasses what I discussed last chapter and adds a few more helpful hints. I'll address each in more detail in a second and then explain how to put this into practice.

> Basic Eating Rules
>
> 1. Eat more frequently
> 2. Eat plenty of lean protein
> 3. Eat a moderate amount of fat at each meal
> 4. Eat plenty of fiber from vegetables, fruits, and unrefined carbohydrates like beans
> 5. Eat moderate amounts of refined carbohydrates such as breads, pasta, rice and grains
> 6. Eat slowly
> 7. Continue to utilize free meals and/or structured refeeds
> 8. Exercise

Eat more frequently

Because of the extremely low-calorie nature of the rapid fat loss plan, it's unlikely that dieters were eating more than 3-4 times per day. It's simply not viable when calories are that low unless you want each meal to be about 3 bites of food.

However, a good bit of research had found that eating more frequently (while splitting your total daily caloric intake) keeps hunger better under control and this is true in both lean and obese individuals (for whom hunger/appetite control can be a real problem). There are a number of reasons for this. Perhaps the biggest one is avoiding extreme hunger which can occur when meals are spaced out too far. This occurs for a number of reasons but decreasing blood glucose is one of them. I'm sure every reader can identify with waiting too long to eat, feeling lightheaded and ending up ravenous at the candy machine.

As an additional benefit, eating smaller meals overall has an effect on the stomach's stretchability, decreasing it over time. Basically, when you eat lots of large meals all of the time, the stomach stretches more. In that the physical stretching of the stomach is one of many signals for fullness, a stomach that is less easily stretched tends to let you know that you're full sooner. Many dieters, coming off of rapid fat loss plan find that they fill up much more quickly with relatively normal sized meals.

Now, I should mention that some earlier research suggested that snacking had the opposite effect, increasing caloric intake and causing weight gain. But this research was really looking at what happens when you add snacks (and I suspect the typical types of junk food snacks) to a normal diet; it wasn't looking at what happens when you split your normal daily food intake into more, smaller meals.

It's the latter goal that I'm describing: splitting your daily food intake into smaller meals. Now, bodybuilders and athletes are used to eating 5-6 (or more) meals per day and take it as part of the price they pay for their sport. But this is often unrealistic for individuals who don't train for a living. Job, life, etc. all get in the way. Consuming 5-6 mini-meals every day simply isn't realistic.

Dieters ending the rapid fat loss plan should maintain at least their previous meal frequency which, as I noted, is probably three to four meals per day. To this they may wish to add smaller snacks for a total of anywhere from four to six "meals" per day. We might figure five "feedings" as a realistic number which would mean breakfast, lunch, and dinner with a couple of small snacks in-between them. I want to make it very clear that all snacks and in-between meals should more or less follow the other rules I'm going to describe as much as possible (getting fiber with a lot of snacks can be a problem but do your best).

That means that an ideal snack should contain protein, a moderate amount of fat, some fiber and the rest. Translation: a plain bagel is not a meal, a piece of fruit is not a meal, and a candy bar surely isn't a meal. A bagel with a bit of mustard, mayo or cheese and some turkey qualifies, a piece of fruit with a glass of low fat milk qualifies, even some of the meal replacement bars (try to pick the ones that have reasonable amounts of protein, carbs and fat) is workable. Would it be ideal to eat a small whole food meal containing protein, fat, fiber and the rest at each meal? Yes. Is that always realistic? No.

Eat plenty of lean protein

As I mentioned last chapter, protein has the greatest effect on blunting hunger, beating out both fat and carbohydrates. Frankly, coming off of a rapid fat loss plan, protein intake should be the least of anybody's concerns since that is most of what they have been eating. Basically, all categories of dieters should simply maintain their protein intake. Category 2 and 3 dieters may wish to increase it slightly if they wish.

Every meal eaten while at maintenance must contain a source of protein and this will go a long way towards keeping caloric intake under control. Protein sources include both those foods listed back in Chapter 8 but can now also include protein that has a higher fat or carbohydrate content. This means some of the leaner cuts of red meat as well as normal dairy such as milk and yogurt (don't forget about the fat intake of such foods). The low-fat cheeses are also fair game although keep in mind the next guideline on fat intake. If you've been eating egg whites at breakfast, you could add a whole egg which will tend to drastically improve the taste.

Eat a moderate amount of fat at each meal

There is a considerable amount of research suggesting that moderate fat diets (20-25% of total calories) are more effective in terms of dietary adherence, as well as being healthier, than either extremely low or extremely high-fat diets. There are a number of reasons for this none of which I'm going to bother getting into.

Now, on the rapid fat loss plan you're already eating a small amount of fat in the form of your EFAs, whether it's the 10 grams per day from either fish oil capsules or liquid fish oil. But, in moving to maintenance, you will need to increase fat intake somewhat at each meal. A reasonable amount would be 10-14 grams per meal as this appears to be optimal in terms of slowing digestion and keeping people full without providing excess calories; smaller snacks should need only half of that, five to seven grams of fat. Ok, now I know that I originally said that you wouldn't have to count or measure stuff but this is a place where I'm going to go back on that.

So you won't skip it, right now I want you go to your kitchen and get out a bottle of vegetable oil (or oil and vinegar salad dressing or something) and a tablespoon measure. Ok, pour the oil into the tablespoon. That's 14 grams of fat right there, that's the maximum you can have at each meal. Right, not very much. Now you see another reason that it's easy to overconsume dietary fat, very little fat contains a ton of calories. I **strongly** advise you to measure your fat intake, at least for a bit. Eyeballing it or estimating it is almost sure to get you into trouble calorie wise.

Now, depending on your other foods choices (especially protein), your meals will probably contain some amount of dietary fat to begin with. This can range from almost none to quite a bit depending on what you eat. Again, this means that you really need to keep track of how much fat you're getting. As a general rule, I'd say this: if your other food choices (such as dairy or other proteins) contain dietary fat, don't add any more to the meal. Odds are there is already enough. If your other foods contain little to no fat (think lean chicken breast or nonfat dairy), you should add a small amount of dietary fat to the meal. Throw some oil and vinegar dressing on your salad or something like that.

I suppose I should mention something about fat sources although this isn't the right book to go into huge details. As noted above, you should already be getting your EFAs from fish oil capsules or liquid. It's nearly impossible to avoid saturated fats if you're eating animal foods although low-fat cheeses and small amounts of butter (a better choice than margarine) are acceptable. That makes olive oil (or high oleic safflower oil for those, like me, who don't like the taste of olive oil) your best bet. So your total daily fat intake at maintenance would come predominantly from monounsaturated fat (olive oil) with additional small amounts of the essential fatty acids and some unavoidable saturated fats.

I'll mention again that the one type of fat you should definitely try to avoid are the trans-fatty acids (aka partially-hydrogenated vegetable oil). These are found in almost all commercial or processed foods.

Eat plenty of fiber from fruits, vegetables and unrefined carbohydrates such as beans

The benefits of fiber go far beyond health; it is a potent aid to both weight loss and maintenance. The reason is that fiber (well, certain types of fiber) keeps food in the stomach longer, promoting fullness. Additionally, that same fiber takes up quite a bit of room in the stomach and the physical stretching of the stomach is one of many signals for fullness. As well, fiber is chewy and takes time to eat; meals high in fiber tend to automatically slow down your eating. This gives your brain time to register that you're full (it typically takes about 20 minutes before your brain realizes that you're full).

Finally, foods high in fiber (fruits, vegetables, naturally occurring carbs like beans and such) are also high in nutrients, both vitamins and minerals that are required for health, as well as a class of nutrients called phytonutrients which are turning out to have numerous health benefits. Once again, your grandmother was right, eat your fruits and vegetables. I should add that some mainstream nutrition types would include the higher fiber grains in this category and this may be true if you're talking about some of the coarser breads. But the more you refine a food, the more fiber you remove and the less nutritious it tends to become. So I'm putting all refined grains in the category of food described in the next section.

Now, while most vegetables (with the exception of the starchy vegetables mentioned previously) have so few calories that they can basically be eaten without limit, this isn't the case for the other foods in this category. The usual issue, as with beans below, has more to do with the toppings people put on top of their veggies; melted cheese is common and many salad dressings contain a considerable amount of calories as carbohydrate, fat, or both.

While difficult, it is conceivable to overeat fruits, especially if you go with stuff like grapes and raisins. Dried fruit is generally a caloric nightmare; by removing the water content, you remove most of the bulk while concentrating the calories. Canned fruit almost always has extra sugar added while fruit juice and offers none of the fullness that eating whole fruit provides. The bulk and fiber has been removed and the calories have been concentrated (i.e. a glass of fruit juice might contain two to three times the caloric content of a piece of fruit without any of the fiber or bulk to actually fill you up).

So go to your produce section in the grocery store and stick with whole fruits and that means eating the skins (where the fiber is) too. As I'll mention below, a single piece of fruit makes a good addition to your normal meals and, unless you go really nuts, you'll be hard pressed to overeat fruit.

The naturally occurring carbohydrate foods such as beans (or legumes, if you prefer) and potatoes can be a bit more problematic. While it's unlikely that most people would drastically overconsume such foods, it is a possibility so be aware. But both are high in fiber (make sure and eat the skin on the potato) and bulk so they will tend to limit their own intake.

Perhaps a bigger issue is what people tend to put on such foods as toppings. A baked potato by itself (or with something like ketchup, my preference, or fat free ranch dressing or salsa) is one thing; a potato smothered in butter and sour cream (how most people eat it) is another entirely. Bean salads are often swimming in oil and people often bury all of the above foods (ok, not fruit) in high fat cheese more often than not.

Finally are nuts which I suppose belong in this category. Frankly, nuts are a bit strange. On the one hand, many nuts contain a good bit of fat and a lot of calories. On the other, they also contain protein and the fat is primarily healthy fat. More interestingly, studies have generally failed to observe the expected weight gain when nuts are given, but nobody is quite sure why.

It might be the thermic effect of the protein, or the metabolic effects of the healthy fats. In any case, although nuts appear to be something of an exception in terms of their caloric content and the weight gain that they cause, simply be aware that it doesn't take a lot of nuts to provide an absolute ton of calories to the diet. If you choose to eat them, they should be measured (similarly to your fat intake).

Eat moderate amounts of starchy or refined carbohydrates

Now the carb freaks and mainstream nutritionists will take issue with what I'm going to write here but that's tough, it's my book. While the dogma about such foods is that they are wonderful for health, impossible to overeat and all that (and this may be true in the artificial world of the lab and under some very specific circumstances), in the real world this just doesn't turn out to be the case.

Many people are easily able to overconsume such foods. And the fact is that they can be somewhat energy dense (meaning they contain a lot of calories in small bulk). If you don't believe me, go get a box of pasta and look at just how little pasta makes a one or three ounce serving.

Now cook it up and compare that to what you probably would typically eat. If you're any kind of normal, you'd probably eat twice or three times the standard "serving" without even noticing. And that's before you add the toppings, which may range from inconsequential like marinara sauce, to the high fat cream sauces and cheese. The same comment goes for rice and many foods in that category, the amount of calories that most people get consuming "typical" portions is massive compared to what an actual serving is supposed to be (based on the nutrition label). Or check most of the commercial cereals sometime, the standard serving and what most people actually eat have nothing in common.

Similarly, in the US especially, the serving sizes of grain-based foods such as bagels and muffins has exploded in recent years. While a bagel or muffin may have only contained a couple of hundred calories in previous years, calorie counts of 400 or more is not uncommon for the supersized versions. Bread in and of itself usually isn't a huge issue, a slice is usually only so large (unless you're eating Texas toast which is huge) and most people won't eat that many slices in a single sitting.

Perhaps a larger problem comes when you add these types of foods to the rest of the modern diet: super high in fat, and low in fiber. Add to that insulin resistance that is common with inactive individuals who are overweight and you start seeing problems. Even marginally refined grains can do bad things to blood glucose and studies are clearly showing that reducing total something called the glycemic load (which is a function of both the amount and type of carbohydrates eaten) and increasing protein intake is better for insulin resistant individuals from a variety of standpoints including blood glucose levels and health.

Now, the point of my comments is not to say that these types of foods are totally off limits (which is an extreme that some nutrition experts reach), simply that such foods can be more problematic than fruits, vegetables and the naturally occurring starches. This is yet another place that I'd highly suggest that you spend a bit of time getting familiar with serving sizes on any of the starch or refined carbohydrate foods that you wish to eat.

Which is to say that serving of pasta or rice or what have you is ok, just don't go crazy with it. Eating a monster bowl of pasta or rice is going to add hundreds and hundreds of calories to your daily intake without you even noticing it. A good rule of thumb might be to limit your starchy carbohydrates at any given meal to the amount that would fit in a cupped palm (just like protein above) or slightly more. This will allow a great deal more food flexibility while still keeping caloric intake under control.

I should mention that some individuals run into problems with even the smallest amount of grains or starches in their diet. These are usually fatter individuals (high end of diet Category 2 or those still in Category 3) who are severely insulin resistant. In that case, grains may simply have to be eliminated completely until body fat levels are reduced and/or activity is increased (regular activity improves insulin sensitivity and carbohydrate tolerance). Which means that fruits, vegetables, and the few naturally occurring starches like potatoes and yams will be the only carbohydrates allowed.

Eat slowly

The idea that eating slowly helps with weight loss and maintenance is yet another place where everyone's grandmother was correct about eating. From a satiation/fullness standpoint, eating more slowly is beneficial. The reason is that there is a delay between eating and when your brain gets the "signal" (which is sent via nerves and chemicals in your bloodstream) that you are full.

On average, the delay is about 20 minutes or so although even this may be impaired in some individuals. The point being that if you eat super quickly, you will tend to eat more than if you take your time. This is one advantage of high-fiber foods, especially salad; they take time to eat. Not surprisingly, a recent study found that people who ate a salad first ate less during the normal meal. Who'd have guessed? I mean other than everybody.

Continue to utilize free meals and/or refeeds

Although the goal of maintenance is, well, maintenance, I still think continuing with free meals as part of your overall structure is a very good idea (for more details see my Guide to Flexible Dieting which talks about flexible vs. rigid dieting). That is, even though the recommendations in this chapter are somewhat free form, there are still restrictions in terms of what you can and can't eat (i.e. you can't eat anything you want in unlimited amounts, that's how you got fat in the first place). Allowing a free meal or two each week can go a long way psychologically to sticking with the other dietary habits you're trying to maintain. The guidelines presented in Chapter 10 should still be followed for free meals.

Occasional refeeds (especially for individuals involved in intense exercise) are also a possibility during maintenance eating, although this is beyond the scope of what I want to cover in this book. If you think you might be in a situation to utilize refeeds during a maintenance phase, drop me an email or see one of my already thoroughly plugged books.

Exercise

I mentioned back in Chapter 7 that a great deal of research has suggested that the primary benefit of exercise is in maintaining weight loss, as it tends not to help much during the diet. There are a few reasons for this. One is that exercise helps to cancel out some of the diet-induced reduction in metabolic rate that can promote weight regain. As well, there tends to be a decrease in resting fat oxidation after the diet, exercise can also correct this defect. Additionally, some research suggests that exercise can increase dietary compliance.

Psychologically, many people seem to link their eating and exercise habits: they tend to be more aware of their eating and strive to eat healthier when they are exercising. I should note that some people take an opposite approach: figuring that they are burning far more calories than they are, they assume that they have earned the double cheeseburger and milkshake after a workout and end up eating too much.

In any event, if you aren't already on an exercise program, while you're moving to maintenance is an excellent time to start. I can't get into all of the details necessary to set up an exercise program in this booklet. You can either check out one of the million and one books on the topic or get my first book The Ketogenic Diet which addresses the issue in some detail. I will say that I think a proper exercise program should contain some mix of resistance exercise (weight training) and cardiovascular or aerobic training.

I should note that the research on this topic tends to find that quite a bit of exercise, about 2500 calories/week is necessary to completely prevent weight regain. Lesser amounts will prevent some of the weight regain but not all of it. Now, this is quite a bit of activity and that is a consideration. To put it into perspective, the average person can burn about 10 calories per minute during a moderate intensity aerobic activity, less if they work at a lower intensity. To burn 2500 calories per week amounts to 400 calories per day if they exercise 6 days per week and progressively more if they exercise fewer days.

This means that about a minimum of 45 minutes (if you're willing to work fairly hard) or up to 90 minutes per day of exercise may be needed to accumulate that 2500 calories/week. Simply keep that in mind when you set up an exercise program. Walking for 20 minutes a few times per week simply isn't going to cut it.

Putting it all together

Ok, so you're coming off of the crash diet, where you've been eating nothing but lots of lean protein, plenty of vegetables, and a little bit of EFAs across 3-4 meals. Frankly, moving from that into the maintenance type of diet described in the above 8 steps is pretty easy. You simply need to add a bit of fat to the meals you're currently eating, some fruit and other naturally occurring carbohydrates to those same meals, add in a moderate amount of refined grains (if you find that you tolerate them well), and another meal/snack or two. With that daily plan, you'd continue with two free meals per week and either continue/increase your current exercise program or embark on one.

Now, once again let me mention that there is both a fast and slow way to move to maintenance and your choice should be made based on the comments I made a couple of chapters back. I'm going to describe the slow method but the end result is basically the same; you would simply add everything in more or less at once.

So the first thing a slow approach individual might do is add a small amount (measured) of dietary fat to each of their three meals along with a piece of fruit. If they were eating egg whites for breakfast, they could simply make one of the eggs a whole egg. Alternately, they could switch from nonfat cheese to one of the low-fat cheeses (which invariably taste and melt much better). A piece of fruit could be added as well. Lunch and dinner would have similar substitutions. Fattier cuts of meats could be chosen (instead of the nonfat choices from Chapter 8) or fat could now be added in the form of a salad dressing (oil and vinegar in measured quantities) to the salads that accompany each meal.

Alternately, the protein choice could remain fat free and some low fat cheese could be sprinkled on the salad (or melted on top of the meat). Dinner would be similar. Adding a starch to the existing meals is a possibility depending on individual preference. A slice or two of a high fiber bread toasted at breakfast, or something similar at lunch and dinner (or a measured amount of pasta or rice) could be added. If you don't want to measure, limit the starch to the amount that would fit in your cupped palm.

If the starches weren't added during the first two days, they could be added at days three and four. If they had already been added, the next addition might be in the form of one or two small snacks in-between the primary meals. Once again, a proper snack should ideally contain protein, fat, a moderate amount of carbs, and some fiber. Usually fiber is the problem with snacks unless you are able to keep vegetables and stuff at work. A small sandwich made out of turkey or chicken breast on high fiber bread with some veggies and mustard would work just fine, a slice of low fat cheese will provide more flavor and a small amount of fat. Again, a piece of fruit and a glass of low fat or 2% milk would be passable as well. A quick alternative would be one of the balanced types of protein bars that contain protein, carbs and some fat.

Once again, the only difference between the slow and fast approach is that the fast approach type of individual would jump straight to a diet consisting of 4-6 small meals each containing protein, vegetables, moderate amounts of fat, some fruit, and a controlled amount of starches (if they are tolerated).

At this point, a very basic maintenance diet would be in place and you'd have fulfilled the 6 major rules above (I don't see that I should have to mention eating slowly again). The only further addition would be to incorporate a free meal once or twice a week, once again using the guidelines set out in Chapter 10. Finally, folks already on an exercise program could now start increasing the amount and frequency of training from the low levels of the rapid fat loss plan; individuals not exercising would be well advised to start a program.

From here on out, it would simply be an issue of playing with food amounts and adjusting intake based on real-world weight or body fat changes. Once again, you can expect to gain a few pounds simply by moving to maintenance, this is simply an issue of increased water and carbohydrate storage. After that, set your weight change window, how much weight gain you'll accept before paying more detailed attention to your diet to head off severe weight regain before it occurs. Three to five pounds in either direction might be a reasonable level with lighter individuals using a smaller window and heavier individuals a larger one.

I'll note again that the above type of freeform approach is not infallible; some folks will find themselves over consuming food/calories if they don't pay at least some attention to detail. In which case the approach described in the next chapter may be a necessary evil. Once again, many people find that a short period measuring everything gives them a far better perspective on what real-world portions are and how much food they should actually be eating. Often then can move back to a more relaxed approach after having going through the pain in the ass that is measuring and counting everything.

94

Moving to Maintenance: Calculation method

So now you've read through some suggestions in the last two chapters on how to move to maintenance without the need to strictly count or control portions. But perhaps you're one of those individuals who want or simply needs more control than that. Or maybe you tried maintaining your weight without tracking portions, it didn't work and you want to calculate, weigh and measure everything for some period of time. This chapter will tell you how to do that. Again, as with several of the previous chapters, all of the calculations I've presented here are done automatically using the online calculator at:

http://rapidfatlosshandbook.com/calculator.php

Let me tell you up front that I'm going to simplify a lot of information in this chapter. Frankly, this chapter and the last three have been a huge headache for me, trying to write something that isn't super complicated but which I am satisfied with in terms of the recommendations I want to give.

The fundamental problem is that I don't think any single diet is appropriate for everyone, what may be ideal depends on such issues as body fat, gender, genetics, food preferences, insulin sensitivity, exercise patterns and a whole host of other topics. When I consult on people's diets, I may have to ask them a dozen or more questions to get a rough idea of what I think might be ideal for them. Even that usually has to be tweaked.

My point being that this chapter is sort of a simplified version of the thought processes I would typically go through in setting up a diet for someone (or myself). It would take the better part of another book (yes, a future book project) to put all of the variables down so I'm sort of copping out here and giving the abbreviated version of how I would approach this topic.

Finally, I want to point out that while you're going to have to do some calculations involving calorie values, you won't be counting calories per se during maintenance. Rather, you'll be counting grams of each nutrient. Which, while the same as counting calories seems not to give people the same headache or anxiety as strict calorie counting. I feel that anybody should be able to look at food label package and pull off the protein, carbs, fat and fiber grams to fill them into daily or meal totals. I hope so anyhow.

Step 1: Determine maintenance calorie levels

The first and most important step in developing a maintenance level diet is to determine maintenance calorie levels. By definition, your maintenance calorie level represents the number of calories per day that you need to maintain your current weight or body fat. Again note that exact body weight/fat maintenance with zero fluctuation is an unrealistic pipe dream. We're going to be a bit more flexible and define maintenance calorie levels as an intake that keeps your body weight/fat within some range.

What this means is that we need to get an estimate of what your total daily calorie expenditure might be. This represents the sum total of calories burned due to basal metabolic rate (BMR), the thermic effect of food (TEF) and the thermic effect of activity (TEA). Lately, researchers have been dividing up the activity component into an exercise component and something they call NEAT (non-exercise activity thermogenesis) which includes all daily movement or activity that isn't formal exercise. Schematically, your total daily energy expenditure could be written as:

$$\text{Total energy expenditure (TEE)} = \text{BMR} + \text{TEF} + \text{TEA} + \text{NEAT}$$

As the name suggests BMR represents the number of calories your body burns at rest, and this typically represents about 60-75% of your total daily energy expenditure. TEF represents the number of calories that are burned in processing food (digestion, storage, etc.). While each of the different nutrients has a different TEF (at least eaten in isolation), on average this amounts to about 10% of your total caloric intake. So if you eat 2000 calories per day, you'll burn about 200 via TEF. TEA represents calories burned during exercise and how much this amounts to can vary drastically from nearly nothing (for someone who is sedentary) to nearly a 100% increase above baseline (for highly active individuals or athletes). Finally is NEAT which, as I mentioned, compromises all daily activities that aren't exercise. Moving around, moving from sitting to standing, fidgeting and others are all encompassed under the heading of NEAT.

While BMR and TEF tend to be fairly consistent, the contribution of activity and NEAT can vary drastically. For example, a sedentary individual may burn effectively zero calories per day in formal exercise while an elite athlete may burn several thousand.

It's turning out that NEAT is very individual and can vary quite a bit; some people burn a lot of calories spontaneously throughout the day just moving around while others don't. This appears to explain some of the rather large differences in weight gain when you overfeed people, some of them ramp up NEAT, burning off a lot of the calories while others do no such thing. The second group gets fat rather readily while the first does not. Unfortunately, NEAT appears to be mostly genetic, nobody has figured out a way to increase it. Your best bet is to simply try and stay active during the day. Sitting all day in front of a computer burns very few calories. Even standing and moving around can contribute rather significantly to overall daily energy expenditure.

In any case, moving forwards I'm going to use some rather standard estimates for each of those three components, adjust it for metabolic rate slowdown due to dieting and use that as an estimate of your maintenance caloric requirement. Unfortunately, there's no easy way to measure NEAT at this point so you'll just have to sort of build it into the estimate you make in a second.

Please note my use of the word estimate, as that is all these values are; do not take them as holy writ. Based on a number of different variables, total daily energy expenditure can have some variance and you will have to make adjustments to your daily caloric intake depending on real world changes in body weight and body fat (which means you need to monitor them to some degree).

Quite simply, if you're regaining weight (this doesn't include the rapid water weight gain that accompanies high carb or salt intakes), you need to cut your calories back a bit; if you're still losing at supposed "maintenance" levels, you need to increase calories slightly.

Depending on activity levels, total daily energy expenditure usually ranges from about 12 calories per pound of body weight for relatively sedentary individuals to 15-16 calories per pound for relatively average activity levels (3-4 hours/week of exercise plus normal daily activity) with extremely active individuals (think endurance athletes training 2 or more hours per day) going up to 20 cal/lb or more.

This means that, on average, a multiplier of 12-16 calories per pound of total body weight is usually about right (with highly trained athletes going higher) to estimate maintenance. Because dieting slows the metabolism somewhat, we're going to adjust that down by about 10% to account for metabolic slowdown giving a range of 11-15 calories per pound or so. Use Table 1 below to select your body weight multiplier. The category descriptions appear below.

Sedentary means no activity other than sitting at a desk (or light household activity). Lightly active would include low intensity aerobic activity. Moderate activity would be either higher intensity aerobic activity or weight training, very active would be a combination of weight training (3+ times/week) and aerobics and extremely active is reserved for athletes in training, individuals training 2 or more hours per day. So use those descriptions as guidelines for picking your body weight multiplier. In general, women (who typically have a lower metabolic rate to start with) should use the lower value, men the higher value.

Table 1 below shows the different multipliers.

Table 1: Body weight multiplier to estimate current maintenance

Description	Body weight multiplier (cal/lb)
Sedentary	10-11
Lightly active	11-12
Moderately active	12-13
Very active	14-15
Extremely active	18-19

Ok, first step, I need you to multiply your current weight in pounds by the above multiplication factor to get your estimated daily maintenance calorie intake per day. Once again, metric readers should multiply their weight in kilograms by 2.2 to get pounds.

_____ * _____ = _____
Weight   Multiplier   Calories/day

This is your estimated caloric requirement per day to maintain you body weight.

The Atwater factors

So what, you ask, are the Atwater factors? They are the values with which I suspect most dieters are already familiar, representing the caloric value of the different nutrients. You'll be using them for the calculations below.. They appear in table 2 below.

Table 2: Atwater factors

Nutrient	Calorie value
Protein	4 calories/gram
Carbohydrate	4 calories/gram
Fat	9 calories/gram
Alcohol	7 calories/gram
Fiber	1.5-2 calories/gram *

*Note that contrary to popular/past belief, the human body does derive a small amount of calories from fiber. Unless fiber intakes are massive (e.g. 50 grams of fiber would yield 75-100 calories), this simply isn't worth worrying about and I'm going to ignore it from here on out. I'm just including it for completeness.

Step 2: Set protein intake

In my opinion, after calories have been set, proper protein intake is the single most important aspect of any diet. This includes fat loss diets, muscle gain diets and maintenance diets. Frankly, no matter what everything else looks like, if protein intake isn't appropriate for the situation, the results will be suboptimal. So before we hassle with carbs or fats, we have to deal with protein.

As I mentioned a chapter or two back, keeping protein higher is turning out to have benefits in terms of weight maintenance in addition to its other benefits and at least one recent study has shown that higher protein intakes after the diet is over help to maintain weight loss. At the very least, it slows weight gain and what weight is regained tends to be LBM. So everybody is going to keep protein intake high.

To simplify things a bit from the chart I gave you back in chapter 8, I'm going to ignore dieting categories here and just focus on activity levels, that will determine how much protein you should be eating at maintenance. In Table 3, you'll see suggested protein intakes in grams per pound of lean body mass.

Table 3: Protein recommendations based on activity levels

Activity level	Protein intake (g/lb)
No activity	0.75
Aerobics only	1.0
Weights *	1.5

Includes folks lifting weights and doing aerobics. For more discussion of the debate over protein requirements for athletes, I'd recommend my new book <u>The Protein Book</u>. Please note that recommendations in that book are based on bodyweight and not LBM for reasons discussed in detail in that book.

Ok, Step 2, you need to multiply your current lean body mass (LBM, not total weight) in pounds by the above value to determine your daily protein intake in grams.

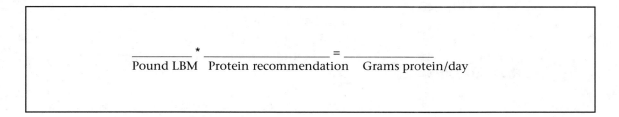

So say you have 125 pounds of LBM and a recommended protein intake of 1 g/lb, that's 125 grams of protein per day.

Now, you're going to multiply total grams of protein by 4 (representing 4 calories per gram which is the Atwater factor) to determine how many calories of protein you'll be eating per day.

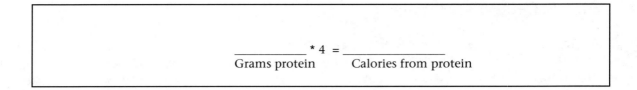

Step 3: Set carbohydrate intake

Ok, figuring out how to set up this part of the diet is probably what gave me the biggest headache of this chapter so I'm going to tell you what the problem is (if I must suffer, you must suffer as well). First and foremost, I don't like diets based on percentages because they have literally no relevance to real human physiology. Telling someone to eat 50% of carbs is meaningless except within the context of total calories so such a recommendation is equally meaningless: 50% could be far too high, far too low, or just right depending on the caloric intake of the individual. Rather, nutrient intakes relative to human needs are better expressed in grams per pound, which is what I did with protein previously and above.

The problem is that, within the context of maintenance, giving an across the board gram per pound recommendation won't work because I can't predict the body weight of my readers. As well, any carbohydrate recommendation I'd give has to be related to both activity, and insulin resistance, along with a few other variables I'd normally take into account. Trying to get that across simplistically still has me stumped so I'm taking a slightly different approach.

One main factor involved in my decision (and my problem) is that I want people consuming at least 100 grams of carbohydrate per day at maintenance. This is especially true for folks who are just doing a 2-week diet break between periods of dieting and is yet another reason that a set gram per pound recommendation wouldn't have worked.

There are a number of reasons I'm picking 100 g/day as the bottom end minimum. First and foremost, at least this many carbs is needed to upregulate thyroid hormone which helps get metabolic rate up again. As well, since leptin levels are sensitive to carbohydrate intake (along with total calories), raising carbs will help to raise leptin further helping to fix metabolic rate. This is especially important for people taking a 2-week diet break but also for people looking at long-term maintenance. Additionally, allowing more carbs in the diet allows for more food variety (while keeping things controlled). This tends to enhance long-term diet adherence (i.e. in the long-term people will quit diets when they get bored of them from an eating perspective).

Finally, 100 g/day will just avoid ketosis, at least in inactive people. Now, this isn't to say that I think being in ketosis is necessarily bad or dangerous but we simply don't know the extended long-term effect of ketosis. Keeping carbs high enough to just avoid ketosis avoids the problem entirely without putting people for whom carb intake can be a problem right back in the same boat that they were in.

Even then, extremely insulin resistant individuals can usually tolerate up to 100 grams per day of carbohydrates though they may need to keep their carb choices limited to vegetables and fruits, no starches. Finally, avoiding ketosis will keep any of your "well meaning" friends or nutrition experts from bitching at you about how unhealthy ketosis is. Your breath and pee won't smell funny anymore either.

So, what I am going to recommend is that everyone start with a baseline carbohydrate intake of 100 grams/day. That's 100 grams regardless of body weight, activity, or anything else. You may end up at a higher carbohydrate intake because of other factors, but you won't ever go lower.

Ok, the next thing is to add an additional amount of carbs by using one of the multipliers below (which are based on the same activity categories that you used in Step one above). So if you're sedentary, your multiplier is zero, if you're lightly active, use 0.5, moderately active, 1, etc. What you're going to do is multiply your current LBM in pounds by that multiplier factor and then add that number to the 100 grams baseline.

Table 4: Carbohydrate recommendations based on activity levels

Description	Body weight multiplier (grams)
Sedentary	0
Lightly active	0.5
Moderately active	1
Very active	1.25
Extremely active	1.5

So let's say you have a LBM of 150 pounds and have an activity level of lightly active. You'd use a multiplier of 0.5 and multiply that by 150 pounds to get 75 grams of carbs. You'd add that to the 100 gram per day baseline for a total carbohydrate intake of 175 grams per day. Or say you have 120 pounds of LBM but are extremely active. You'd multiply 120 pounds by 1.5 to get 180 grams and you'd add that to the baseline value of 100 grams for a total of 280 grams of carbohydrate per day. Clearly anyone who is in the sedentary activity level regardless of LBM will be eating only the baseline 100 grams per day of carbs. Recommendations appear in table 4 below.

Ok, next step.

_____*_____ = _____ + 100 g = _____
LBM in pounds Multiplier Grams carbs   Total daily carbs

As well, just as you did for protein, you're now going to multiply the total grams of carbs by 4 (for 4 calories per gram) to get the total number of carbohydrate calories you'll be eating each day.

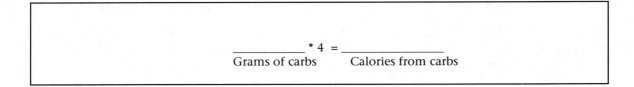

Step 4: Set fat intake

I promise, you're almost done. The last calculation is to determine daily fat intake by subtracting the number of calories you're getting from protein and carbs from your daily total. Basically, fat intake is simply used as a caloric buffer to make up the rest of your daily calories. So first you need to determine how many calories from you'll be eating by subtracting the number of calories from protein and carbs from your daily total.

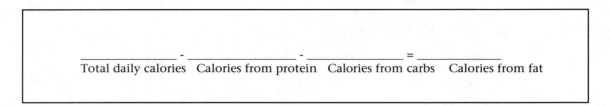

Finally, you will *divide* the total number of fat calories by 9 (representing 9 calories per gram) to get grams of fat per day.

_____ / 9 = _____
Calories from fat   Grams of fat

A note on fiber

I should mention fiber for completeness. As discussed in the previous 2 chapters, maintaining a high fiber intake (by eating vegetables, fruits and even the higher fiber grains) should be an important part of any diet, including a maintenance diet. Since you were consuming lots of veggies already on the PSMF, all you really need to do is keep up that intake and, as discussed last chapter, add fruits and moderate amounts of higher fiber starches and grains. If you do that, fiber intake should be a non-issue; you'll be getting plenty automatically.

What I occasionally see happening (and often do myself) is that once people are allowed to eat carbohydrates other than the high fiber ones (vegetables), they tend to quit eating vegetables. That is, when you constrain people to only eating vegetables and fruits, that's what they'll eat; when you allow them starches, they forget about the good stuff and eat nothing but starches. Don't do this.

Step 5: Putting it all together

Ok, step 5 is simply to gather all of the values from above for easy reference. So take your protein grams from step 2, carb grams from step 3 and fat grams from step 4 and write them below. That's your maintenance diet to be consumed on a daily basis.

Grams protein per day (from Step 2): _____

Grams carbs per day (from Step 3): _____

Grams fat per day (from Step 4): _____

These values would more or less be divided up across however many meals you're choosing to eat (see Chapter 13 for some comments on meal frequency and snacking). As I've mentioned, bodybuilders and athletes would typically try to divide those nutrients relatively evenly across their five to six (or more) meals but this may not be realistic for everyone. As discussed in Chapter 13, three larger meals with one or more snacks throughout the day may be more attainable for people who can't dedicate their lives to training and eating.

However, and I want to make this point as clearly as possible (this is why I suggested everyone read the previous 2 chapters), any meal or snack should ideally still contain some amount of all the nutrients (and ideally some fiber though this can be a problem). Basically, you should follow the same basic guidelines as described in the past 2 chapters, the only real difference is that you're now keeping more accurate track of your food intake.

In general, I find it best if people pick their protein source first. The reason is that proteins typically either contain some fat (most meats) or carbohydrates (dairy and such). Meaning that you have to figure those values into the overall meal calculation. You can use the chart back in Chapter 8 to get an idea of the amounts of protein you'll need at each meal to meet your goals.

Next, ensure your vegetable intake. Think salad, or veggies in that morning omelet, or on your sandwich or in a salad or what have you. Even rigid calorie counter don't need to worry too much about measuring vegetable intake, you'd have to eat a metric ton of them for it to add many calories. The only exceptions, again, are the starchy vegetables carrots, peas, corn, potatoes, etc. which can add a lot of carbohydrate calories to a meal.

Frankly, the bigger issue with salads is usually dressing, as most contain a lot of sugar and fat. The common dieting approach is to get the dressing on the side (and try to pick either a low-cal or low fat version) and dip your fork into it. You'll end up using a lot less of it than if you just try to bury your salad in it. Many find that the lower fat versions of salad dressing taste just as good while saving them a tremendous number of calories each day.

Fruit would be next and would be applied to your total carbohydrate intake. An average piece of fruit (e.g. apple or banana) will contain about 20-25 grams of carbs or so (this will, of course, vary with the size). With fruits like grapes or raisins, you'll have to look it up and track it yourself, just be aware that a rather small amount of food can add up to a lot of calories if you're not careful.

As mentioned in the last chapter, I think dried fruit is a poor choice; a very small volume can contribute a ton of calories. Fruit juice, as stated, is a horrid choice as far as I'm concerned: it's a glass of concentrated sugar water without any of the fiber or bulk that makes whole fruits such a good food choice.

Next, assuming you have any carbohydrate grams left, you can add a starch if you want. If you're really intolerant to them for some reason, a second piece of fruit can work instead. Starches and whole grains can add a surprising number of carbohydrate calories (especially rice, pasta and the new monster bagels) so read the labels, get out the measuring spoons and figure it out. To give you a few ideas, a typical slice of bread has about 15 grams of carbs, a glass of milk or cup of yogurt about 12, a small baked potato about 25 grams.

Finally, if you haven't used it up with the other foods, you can add your dietary fat. Note again that the foods you've already chosen, even if technically no-fat will have a little bit. If you choose a fattier cut of meat or low-fat or 2% dairy, you've already gotten some as well. But whatever you have left can then be added. Oil and vinegar salad dressings work well and controlled amounts of other fats (e.g. mayo, peanut butter) are acceptable.

As mentioned last chapter, it would be ideal to focus on monounsaturated fats for most of your additional fat intake. You'll get sufficient saturated fats unless you really go out of your way to choose nothing but nonfat meats and dairy and you should still be covering your essential fatty acid requirements from either fish oil capsules or liquid fish oil.

What I personally have found works best is this: take the time to sit down and come up with what are essentially modular meals. That is, pick a protein, pick your veggies, add your carbs (fruit/starches), then your fat. Work them out so that they conform to your meal or snack goals. Most people tend to eat more or less the same day in day out, especially if you're looking at the breakfast or lunch meals (dinner tends to be the most variable).

If you have to eat out a lot, figuring out what places allow you to meet your nutritional requirements most easily may be a good thing to do; most places have calorie counts for their foods. For smaller snacks, either work out some mini-meals or find pre-made food bars which meet your requirements for each nutrient.

Although this can be an initial hassle, you'll eventually reach a point where you can just sort of rotate meals, as they will be more or less interchangeable. After some time measuring everything, you'll also have a pretty good idea of how to eyeball your foods and get within shooting distance.

Oh yeah, just as with the non-counting approach to maintenance, I still suggest 1 or 2 free meals per week, even if you're counting calories. Hell, just go read the past chapter, everything I said there applies, you're just counting things now.

Making adjustments

As I mentioned at the first of the chapter, the values I gave for nutrient recommendations are nothing but estimates upon estimates and should not be taken as anything more than that. At the end of the day, real world changes in your body composition, weight or fat (again this necessitates regular monitoring) should be the ultimate determinant. If your weight is slowly climbing, you need to cut your food intake back or increase your activity.

Given the choice of the three nutrients, I'd generally suggest that you cut back your carbohydrate (starches and grains, fruits if you have to) intake a bit. Cutting back fat slightly is another option although very low fat diets tend to backfire, as I've mentioned, leaving people hungrier at the end of the day. Under no circumstances do I think you should cut your protein, vegetable or EFA intake.

If you're still in a situation where your weight is moving down slowly, well, you have a couple of options. If further weight loss is your goal, you can just run with it. If you are more interested in weight stability for the time being, increase your food intake slightly. Carbohydrates or fats would be the best bet here since both protein and fat intake should already be at an acceptable level.

In neither case should huge changes be necessary or made. If your weight is gradually creeping up, try cutting 100-200 calories out of your diet. That would mean either a 25-50 gram reduction in carbohydrates or about a 10-20 gram reduction in fat. Same for weight loss but in reverse, add a couple of hundred calories per day until weight stabilizes. This is discussed in more detail in the final chapter.

Back To Dieting

Ok, one more chapter and we're done. The previous three chapters dealt with how to move to maintenance using one of two different approaches: a non-calculating method (Chapter 12 and 13) and a pain in the ass method where you calculate and measure your food (Chapter 14). As I mentioned previously, both approaches were also valid for dieters who were simply taking a 2-week diet break as described back in Chapter 10.

That group of individuals, who was simply taking a diet break, will be moving back into dieting (where fat/weight loss is the explicit goal) and I want to make a few comments about that. Basically, such folks will diet down for a while, take a break, diet down further, take another break, diet some more, until they reach their goal.

At some point, obviously, they'll move into maintenance just as described in the previous chapters. I think this approach is better almost without exception (the exception is dieters under a specific time frame) and wish more people would do it.

By definition, any diet that generates fat or weight loss must contain fewer calories than your maintenance level. Which means that, also by definition, if you have been eating at maintenance for the past 2 weeks (or longer if that's the case), you need to be eating less than you are now if you want to generate weight or fat loss. Alternately, you can increase your activity while eating the same amount. Since the increase activity will increase your maintenance caloric requirement, you'd now be eating below maintenance.

This means that regardless of what you do, you're going to have to readjust either food intake or activity to get weight and fat loss moving again. Simplistically, at least within the context of this booklet, there are two different approaches I expect people to take in moving back into weight/fat loss.

I want to mention as well, that with the exception of extreme approaches like the rapid fat loss program, a 1-2 pound week fat/weight loss is about all that can realistically be expected with a more moderate or traditional type of calorically restricted diet. Extremely large or fatter individuals will often lose somewhat more (maybe 3-4 pounds) but lighter individuals should be more than happy with a consistent weekly weight/fat loss of 1-2 pounds. Many, especially lighter females, will have to settle for less, ½ pound per week is often the fastest the fat will come off.

Two different groups

Ultimately I guess there are probably two groups of folks who I need to address in this book. The first group, who would only be in dieting Category 2 or 3, may wish to move back to another stretch of the PSMF to generate more rapid weight/fat losses (I strongly discourage Category 1 dieters from even considering this unless, for some reason, it was absolutely necessary).

The folks doing another stint on the rapid fat loss plan shouldn't need much in the way of guidelines. Just go back and recalculate your food intake using your new weight (and possibly new dieting Category) as described in this booklet and get to it. Don't forget to include the free meals, refeeds or another full break as discussed in Chapter 10.

The second group is the one that I mentioned way early in the book, who want to use a PSMF to kickstart their weight/fat loss efforts (and maybe fix some eating habit problems) and then move into a more moderate or traditional type of diet. That's the group I want to address here.

The typical approach to calorie restriction

A typical approach to weight loss would be to recommend some fixed calorie level to everyone, although usually men and women are given different recommendations (e.g. 1200 and 1500-1800 cal/day for women and men respectively). I consider this approach fairly ludicrous.

For those of you who read the last chapter, it should be clear that your maintenance calorie requirements depend on both activity level and body weight. Telling two different men (let's say that one is 150 pounds and highly active and the other is 400 pounds and inactive) that they should eat the same number of calories for weight loss is either ignorance or just laziness on the part of the author. Perhaps a bit of both.

Another typical approach would be to recommend that everyone reduce their daily caloric intake by anywhere from 500-1000 calories per day, depending on whether they want a 1 or 2 pound weight loss per week. That is, as the math and logic go, since one pound of fat contains 3,500 calories, if you eat 500 calories/day less, you will lose one pound of fat per week; 1000 calories per day less and you will lose two. It never works out that perfectly (people never seem to lose exactly the predicted amount of fat per week that the numbers indicate) for reasons unimportant to this book.

Rather I want to point out the problem with giving an absolute caloric reduction for everyone. Again, the issue has to do with body weight, activity and maintenance calorie intakes. If a light female, who may have a maintenance requirement of about 1700 calories per day, reduces her food intake by 500 calories, she's at 1200 calories for the day. If she reduces her total food intake by 1000, she's at 700 cal/day. This is not a lot of food. By the same token, a large male with a maintenance intake of 3500 calories is still at a rather hefty 3000 cal per day with a 500 cal per day reduction. He'll be at 2500 cal per day if he reduces his daily food intake by 1000 calories. Basically, a flat daily caloric reduction doesn't take into account the variance in estimated intake: lighter individuals end up taking a much larger drop (as a percentage of their maintenance) than heavier individuals. They also end up at a far lower absolute value of food intake.

I don't like either of the above methods. The first is simply silly; no single caloric recommendation can possibly apply across the board. Even if you split it up into male and female recommendations, it's still absurd to think that all females should eat the same number of calories regardless of weight or activity. The second is equally problematic, as the same absolute caloric reduction tends to have drastically different affects on food intake depending on the person's current maintenance needs.

My preferred method

My preferred method, as I originally described in my first book The Ketogenic Diet, is to simply reduce food intake relative to your current daily maintenance. This means that any reductions are made relative to what you actually need to eat (or are currently eating, assuming your weight is stable). So the person eating only 1700 calories/day has a smaller food reduction than someone eating 3000 calories/day. Since I've described two different approaches for moving to maintenance, I have to make comments for each.

For folks using the non-measurement method described in Chapters 12 and 13, that would basically mean just reducing their food intake slightly from what they are eating now. My primary recommendation would be to cut back on concentrated starches first (which tend to contribute the most calories without doing a great job of filling people up), fat intake can be reduced slightly (I wouldn't go less than one half tablespoon or 7 grams of fat per meal, though) or some of the fruit can be dropped out. At no point should protein or vegetable intake be reduced.

That small reduction in food intake would be maintained for a few weeks and then the person would look at their weight/fat loss. As above, short of extreme approaches, a realistic weekly fat loss is usually 1-2 pounds. Lighter women may be lucky to get 1 pound/week but heavier/fatter individuals can often get more. But based on real world changes, further reductions could be made based on what is actually happening. So if you're losing less than one pound per week on average, you can reduce your food intake (or increase activity) slightly more until you hit the sweet spot.

If someone were calculating nutrients as per the last chapter, I'd have them reduce their food intake by 10-20% per day from what they are eating at maintenance. So if they had a maintenance level of 3000 calories per day based on activity and body weight, they'd reduce by 300-600 calories per day. If they had a maintenance level of 1700 cal per day, they'd reduce by 170-340 calories per day. Which means that they have to go recalculate their carb and fat intakes based on that change to their daily caloric intake.

As always, protein intake stays the same, with the adjustment coming to carbohydrate and fat intake. As above, it may simply be easiest for dieters to reduce their concentrated carbohydrate (starch) intakes to achieve the calorie reduction. Or use some mix of carbohydrate and fat reduction.

After adjusting their food intake, they'd stay at that level for 2-3 weeks and track changes in body composition. Based on real world changes, they'd make the following adjustments. The adjustment schema I use appears below with a few notes of explanation below that.

Table 1: Weekly average fat loss and how to adjust daily calories

Average weekly fat loss	Change to caloric intake
Less than 1 lb/week	Reduce calories by 10%
1-1.5 lb/week	No change
2+ pounds/week:	
Category 1 dieters involved in heavy training	
No performance loss	No change
Performance loss	Increase calories by 10%
Category 2 and 3 dieters	No change

The first two situations should be fairly clear to most people. If you're losing less than one pound per week on average, and you're not an extremely light female, you need to cut calories further; another 10% reduction would be appropriate. Then maintain that for 2-3 weeks and remeasure body composition.

Anybody who is losing a consistent 1-1.5 pounds per week is basically in the sweet spot as far as I'm concerned. They shouldn't change a thing. If they are in dieting Category 2 or 3, they can consider a further 10% calorie reduction to see if they can achieve a slightly higher weekly fat loss. Frankly, anyone achieving 1-1.5 pounds/week on a consistent basis is doing really well.

The most complicated situation, as the chart above indicates is whether or not a loss of greater than 2 pounds per week (again, this is under moderate dieting conditions) is cause for alarm. Basically, it depends on the circumstances.

A Category 2 or 3 dieter may have no problem losing that much weight weekly and probably shouldn't adjust calories. The real issue is for Category 1 dieters, especially if they are involved in high intensity activity, a weekly two pound weight loss often signals LBM loss. Category 1 dieters involved in heavy training should use their performance or strength as the deciding factor. If they are losing 2 pounds per week and NOT losing strength or seeing a decrement in performance, they are probably ok. But they should be very alert to the possibility of overtraining, performance loss, and muscle loss. If strength in the gym or athletic performance is showing a large drop, Category 1 dieters should increase calories by 10% to reduce the rate of weight loss.

A couple of comments about the above chart

I should mention that, rather than reducing caloric intake by 10%, it is also possible to increase activity (via exercise) instead. So let's assume that someone is currently eating 2000 calories/day and losing less than one pound per week. If, for some reason, they didn't want to decrease their calories (by 10% or 200 calories), they could increase their activity level to burn an additional 200 calories instead (this would require anywhere from 10-30 minutes of added exercise per day depending on the intensity). By the same token, if someone were losing too quickly, rather than increase their food intake by 10%, they could reduce the amount of activity they were doing.

I bring this up because dieters often run into situations where further reductions in calories are simply unrealistic; this is especially true when caloric intakes get very low. In those situations, adding activity may be the only way to create a suitable deficit. This is often true for women and lighter men; their daily caloric requirements are so low to begin with that there is a very real limit to how far food intake can be reduced. They are probably better off increasing activity in terms of long-term diet success.

I should mention that it is exceedingly rare for fat loss to occur in a linear or nonstop fashion. Rather, it's extremely common for stalls of several weeks to occur followed by major drops in scale weight and changes in appearance, seemingly overnight. Empirically, these drops often occur after performing a structured refeed. My guess is that it has to do with screwy water balance on a diet but I can't really support that with any hard data. Just be aware of it, especially when you're wondering whether or not you should make adjustments below.

I bring this up for the following reason: let's say that you've made an alteration to your food intake and stayed there for 2-3 weeks. Now it looks like nothing is happening. By the above chart, you need to reduce food intake (or increase activity), right? Well, maybe. It may very well be that, given another week (or by incorporating a structured refeed), things will start moving. I can't give any really super accurate guidelines for what you should do; simply be aware that an apparent zero change over a few weeks may suddenly become visible rather rapidly. Again, I can't explain why it works this way, only that it does.

A final note about moderate dieting

As with the crash diet, it is more than possible to diet for too long at a stretch. Frankly, I think that most people do exactly that. Basically, they stay in diet mode forever when they'd do better, in the long run, breaking up their dieting phases. As well, and as discussed in much more detail in <u>A Guide to Flexible Dieting</u>, incorporating free meals, refeeds and full diet breaks still applies to more traditional/moderate dieting. The only difference, really, is that the full diet breaks don't need to come quite as often.

For the average Category 1 dieter, I feel that 4-6 weeks of moderate dieting is about the maximum (occasionally, 8 weeks can be acceptable). After that, a 2-week diet break should be undertaken as described in the past chapters. If further fat loss is necessary, they can move back into moderate dieting. As well, and in contrast to the rapid fat loss plan. Category 1 dieters should incorporate free meals once or twice a week. Structured refeeds should also be used but the details are beyond the scope of this booklet. You'll have to buy either A Guide To Flexible Dieting or my Ultimate Diet 2.0 for the details.

Category 2 dieters may diet somewhere between 6-12 weeks or so before going on a full diet break. Shorter dieting spans are also acceptable but only if weight/fat regain is avoided during the diet break. The same guidelines for free meals, one or two per week applies from Chapter 10. Category 2 dieters may consider a structured refeed of 1 full day roughly every 10-14 days although some of that will depend on training intensity, volume and frequency.

Finally, Category 3 dieters are still in a position to diet for the longest stretch without a break. 12-16 weeks would be an appropriate amount before doing another full diet break. As with Category 2 dieters, they may consider shorter dieting periods but only if they aren't regaining too much weight or fat during the break. Free meals are the same as always at two per week. Finally, refeeds may be considered at a frequency of 5 hours once every 14-21 days. Once again, see my Guide to Flexible Dieting for all of the details and guidelines for refeeds.

Appendix 1: BMI and Body fat charts

As discussed in the main text of this book, BMI can be used to roughly estimate body fat percentage and readers can use Table 1, 2 and 3 (or the online calculator) to first estimate BMI (Table 1 and 2) and then estimate body fat percentage (Table 3). I want to make it abundantly clear again that active individuals should not and can not use this method to estimate body fat percentage, they must find another method. As a final reminder, the online calculator will give you both BMI and estimated body fat percentage:

http://www.rapidfatlosshandbook.com/calculator.php

Table 1: BMI Chart Part 1 (Short-folks)

Feet		4'10	4'11	5'0	5'1	5'2	5'3	5'4	5'5	5'6	5'7
Meters		1.47	1.5	1.52	1.55	1.57	1.60	1.63	1.65	1.68	1.70
Lb	Kg										
100	45	21	20	20	19	18	18	17	17	16	16
110	50	23	22	22	21	20	20	19	18	18	17
120	55	25	24	23	23	22	21	21	20	19	19
130	60	27	26	25	25	24	23	22	22	21	20
140	64	29	28	27	26	26	25	24	23	23	22
150	68	31	30	29	28	28	27	26	25	24	24
160	73	33	32	31	30	29	28	28	27	26	25
170	77	36	34	33	32	31	30	29	28	28	27
180	82	38	36	35	34	33	32	31	30	29	28
190	86	40	38	37	36	35	34	33	32	31	30
200	91	42	40	39	38	37	35	34	33	32	31
210	95	44	43	41	40	39	37	36	35	34	33
220	100	46	45	43	42	40	39	38	37	36	35
230	105	48	47	45	44	42	41	40	39	37	36
240	109	50	49	47	45	44	43	41	40	39	38
250	114	53	51	49	47	46	45	43	42	41	39
260	118	54	53	51	49	48	46	45	43	42	41
270	123	57	55	53	51	50	48	47	45	44	42
280	127	59	57	55	53	51	50	48	47	45	44
290	132	61	59	57	55	53	52	50	48	47	46
300	136	63	61	59	57	55	53	51	50	48	47
310	141	65	63	61	59	57	55	53	52	50	49
320	145	67	65	62	60	58	57	55	53	52	50
330	150	69	67	65	62	60	59	57	55	53	52
340	155	71	69	67	65	63	61	59	57	55	54
350	159	73	71	68	66	64	62	60	58	57	55
360	164	76	73	71	68	66	64	62	60	58	57
370	168	77	75	72	70	68	66	64	62	60	58
380	173	80	77	75	72	70	68	66	64	62	60
390	177	82	79	76	74	71	69	67	65	63	61
400	182	84	81	78	76	73	71	69	67	65	63

Table 2: BMI Chart Part 2 (Tall folks)

Feet		5'8	5'9	5'10	5'11	6'0	6'1	6'2	6'3	6'4
Meters		1.73	1.75	1.78	1.80	1.83	1.85	1.88	1.91	1.93
Lb	Kg									
100	45	15	15	14	14	14	13	13	13	12
110	50	17	16	16	15	15	15	14	14	13
120	55	18	18	17	17	16	16	15	15	15
130	60	20	19	19	18	18	17	17	16	16
140	64	21	21	20	20	19	18	18	18	17
150	68	23	22	22	21	20	20	19	19	18
160	73	24	24	23	22	22	21	21	20	20
170	77	26	25	24	24	23	22	22	21	21
180	82	27	27	26	25	24	24	23	23	22
190	86	29	28	27	27	26	25	24	24	23
200	91	30	30	29	28	27	26	26	25	24
210	95	32	31	30	29	29	28	27	26	26
220	100	34	33	32	31	30	29	28	28	27
230	105	35	34	33	32	31	31	30	29	28
240	109	37	35	34	34	33	32	31	30	29
250	114	38	37	36	35	34	33	32	31	31
260	118	40	38	37	36	35	34	33	33	32
270	123	41	40	39	38	37	36	35	34	33
280	127	43	41	40	39	38	37	36	35	34
290	132	44	43	42	41	39	38	37	36	35
300	136	46	44	43	42	41	40	38	37	36
310	141	47	46	45	43	42	41	40	39	38
320	145	49	47	46	45	43	42	41	40	39
330	150	50	49	47	46	45	44	42	41	40
340	155	52	50	49	48	46	45	44	43	42
350	159	53	52	50	49	48	46	45	44	43
360	164	55	53	52	50	49	48	46	45	44
370	168	56	55	53	52	50	49	48	46	45
380	173	58	57	55	54	52	51	49	48	47
390	177	59	58	56	54	53	51	50	49	47
400	182	61	59	58	56	54	53	52	50	49

To determine BMI, locate your height on the top row (the top value is height in feet and inches, the bottom is meters) and then cross-reference it with weight on the left hand column (left most column is weight in pounds, right column is weight in kilograms).

So an individual who is 5'0" (1.52 meters) tall and 150 pounds (68 kilograms) will have a BMI of 28. If your weight falls in between two values, simply take the halfway value of the two. So a 5'2" (1.57 meter) individual weighing 165 pounds (~75 kg) would estimate their BMI halfway between the 160 and 170 lb values of 26 and 28 to get a BMI of 27.

Once you have your BMI, use Table 3 to get a rough estimate of your body fat percentage. Once again please note that this is only an estimate and that active and/or athletic individuals cannot use this method, as it will drastically misestimate them. The equations also tend to be less accurate at either extreme (extremely lean or extremely fat) of body fat percentage. But, once again, it is for inactive people only.

Table 3: BMI and Body fat percentage

BMI	Female BF%	Male BF%	BMI	Female BF%	Male BF%
13	13.5	You are dead	27	34.5	21.5
14	15	You are dead	28	36	23
15	16.5	You are dead	29	37.5	24.5
16	18	5	30	39	26
17	19.5	6.5	31	40.5	27.5
18.5	21	8	32	42	29
19	22.5	9.5	33	43.5	30.5
20	24	11	34	45	32
21	25.5	12.5	35	46.5	33.5
22	27	14	36	48	35
23	28.5	15.5	37	49.5	36.5
24	30	17	38	51	38
25	31.5	18.5	39	52.5	39.5
26	33	20	40	54	41

Note: If your BMI is over 40, add 1.5% body fat for each BMI point.

116

My Other Books

Depending on what your typical reading materials are, you may or may not be familiar with my other books (I mean beyond my endless mentioning of them in the text of this booklet) so I thought I'd bring them to your attention in case you are at all interested in what else I have written. All of them can be ordered through my website at http://www.bodyrecomposition.com

The Protein Book: A Complete Guide for the Athlete and Coach (Published 2007)

Similar to my first book on the ketogenic diet, The Protein Book is a comprehensive look at the topic of dietary protein for athletes. Every topic from basic protein metabolism, protein requirements, nutrient timing around training and supplements is discussed. As well, each whole food protein and protein powder is examine in terms of its pros and cons for athletes. Of course, how to put all of the information together for different kinds of athletes (strength/power, endurance, physique) is included. The book is over 200 pages and includes over 500 scientific references.

A Guide to Flexible Dieting (Published 2005)

Also mentioned repeatedly in this booklet, this book expands on the ideas of free meals, refeeds and the diet break that are mentioned in this booklet. It doesn't describe any specific diet plan; dealing primarily with the idea of rigid versus flexible dieting.

The Ultimate Diet 2.0 (Published 2004)

I must have mentioned my UD2 a dozen or more times in the text of this booklet. The UD2 is an updating of the original Ultimate Diet that was written nearly 20 years ago. It is a diet for hardcore dieters who are already very lean (12-15% body fat or lower for men) and who want to get even leaner without losing any muscle.

The Ketogenic Diet: A Complete Guide for the Dieter and Practitioner (Published 1998).

This was my first project and it's a monster. It's 325 pages of information dense text with over 600 scientific references. To say that it is the be-all, end-all guidebook for low-carbohydrate/ketogenic diets is an understatement. There's really no other book in its category. I should note that it is written in a very different style than this booklet or my others; it's somewhat dry and very technical. It covers nutritional and exercise physiology and gives recommendations for three different types of low-carbohydrate diets, as well as sample exercise programs from beginner to advanced. It is really for the hardcore low-carbohydrate dieter who truly wants to know everything that is going on in their body when they are in ketosis.